Good health—is there a choice?

Fifth Kellogg Nutrition Symposium

Good health—is there a choice?

Edited by

P. H. Fentem

First published 1981 by
THE MACMILLAN PRESS LTD
London and Basingstoke
Companies and representatives throughout the world

ISBN 0 333 31139 6

A/613

Reproduced from copy supplied
printed and bound in Great Britain
by Billing and Sons Limited
Guildford, London, Oxford, Worcester

Contents

The Contributors

MRS. L. BAILEY BSc
Community Education Section,
The Open University

A.E. BENDER BSc, PhD, FIFST
Professor of Nutrition and Dietetics,
Queen Elizabeth College,
University of London

P.H. FENTEM MSc, MB, ChB
Professor of Physiology,
University of Nottingham
Medical School

DR A. MARYON DAVIS MSc, MRCP, MFCM
Assistant Medical Officer,
The Health Education Council

DR T.W. MEADE BM, FRCP
Director,
MRC Epidemiology and Medical
  Care Unit,
Northwick Park Hospital

DR R.G. WHITEHEAD PhD, MA, FIBiol
Director,
Dunn Nutritional Laboratory,
University of Cambridge and
  Medical Research Council

DR A. YOUNG BSc, MRCP
Clinical Lecturer in
  Rehabilitation Science,
Nuffield Department of
  Orthopaedic Surgery,
University of Oxford

Sir George YOUNG Bt, MP
Parliamentary Under Secretary
  of State,
Department of Health and
  Social Security

Foreword

The selection of *Good Health – Is There A Choice?* as the theme for the Fifth Kellogg Nutrition Symposium reflected the growing belief that people could lead healthier lives if they chose to do so. It was felt that the contributors should examine two principal areas – 'exercise' and 'eating' – and by their expertise inspire informed discussion amongst those engaged in promoting better health measures and by the public at large. Without exception the speakers at this symposium achieved their objectives and all the participants gained much benefit.

In publishing these proceedings we consider that we have made a useful addition to the advisory literature which is now being published by the Health Education Council, The British Nutrition Foundation and other organisations for the people of Great Britain. Such publications do enable the practising reader to make correct decisions about those factors that influence the quality of life and health.

Understanding nutrition and its relationship to health will strongly influence the selection of sensible meals. The choice of correct meals will enable the body to function more efficiently through proper energy control and the provision of a balanced intake of essential nutrients with an adequate level of dietary fibre. Linked with these considerations is the significance of undertaking regular and appropriate exercise. Sensible exercise keeps the body working efficiently, helps weight control and exercises the heart. All these factors are becoming more widely known. Together with a few simple health guidelines they can make life more enjoyable through the life span.

In concert with all those who contributed to the success of this symposium we believe that anyone concerned with the issues of health education will find the book helpful. Indeed it is hoped that the book will be even more widely read than just by those engaged in education.

GOOD HEALTH – IS THERE A CHOICE?

The Kellogg Company of Great Britain Limited wishes to express most sincere thanks and appreciation to all the authors and those who assisted in the organisation of this symposium.

W.D.B. HAMILTON
Director of Scientific Affairs – European Division
Kellogg Company of Great Britain Limited

1
The choice is yours

SIR GEORGE YOUNG

May I first congratulate you on choosing as your theme for the symposium 'Good Health — Is There a Choice?'. It seems to me to be a most appropriate theme at a time when there is undoubtedly a growing awareness that problems in many areas of our lives — health, law and order, wealth creation — can only be tackled successfully if choice is exercised and those concerned understand the issues and consequences of their actions and voluntarily decide to act responsibly. This seems to me to be a most encouraging reaction to the alternative and somewhat fatalist view that the individual is powerless and should reconcile himself to whatever fate has in store for him. As Bernard Levin wrote in the *Times*:

> 'We are, ultimately, responsible for what we are, and we cannot escape that responsibility. And if we believe those who tell us that we can, that nothing is our fault, that we are products of what was done to us by 'society' (or, in full, 'capitalist society'), that we can act as we please and escape the consequences by pleading force majeure ("I had no more choice of action than any man who acts in accordance with his beliefs . . . "), then we not only damn ourselves, but go another step along the road to the damnation of our entire world'.

That seems to me to sum up a great deal of the question. But it also poses another one — whose choice? Just the individual, or does the Government have a role to play here?

Government should clearly prevent poisonous substances from being sold, but how much further should it go? What is the right balance of responsibility in a free society between Government and individual?

The critics of placing more emphasis on *individual* responsibility will allege that the Government is seeking a way of getting prevention on the cheap and is

1

opting out of its responsibilities. I don't see it that way. Of course, every health minister would like to see the nation healthier, and to that end we have all pumped thousands of millions of pounds into the NHS. That solution is now producing diminishing returns, ever more expensive to secure. The big improvements will not come from traditional curative medicine, but from less traditional preventive medicine and, whereas the first is certainly the responsibility of Government, the second is less obviously so.

We must also have regard, particularly in a Conservative Government, to the limits of action that Government can take in pressing the claims of preventive action on the public and compelling people to alter their lifestyle. We can assess what preventive measures can have positive health benefits, and it is right that a Government must encourage the dissemination of this information either through the medium of the Health Education Council or by way of Government publications, or through speeches such as this, but we must be alert to the danger of pressing the public too far to the extent that the good effects are nullified by a public resentment at 'Government interference'. Government interference in all our lives has increased considerably, rightly so in many areas where there are complex social and economic problems. However, there have been indications that the threshold of public acceptance of Government 'nannying' has been reached – and in some instances passed – in many areas of our lives. I would certainly not want us to press too hard and so put in danger the goodwill and the splendid work that is being done in preventive work.

So Governments do have a part to play in the matter of choices but it is the individual who has the ultimate responsibility for the maintenance of good health as it is he and not 'the Government' that makes choices in his personal lifestyle. The Government can help him to make informed choices. We approach this by funding the Health Education Council which is responsible for national health education campaigns and by Government publications on Prevention and Health and on health aspects of nutritional issues.

The Health Education Council has carried out a number of campaigns over recent years covering such matters as family planning, correct exercise and diet, respect for medicines and warnings against cigarette smoking. Perhaps the most widely known campaign is 'Look After Yourself', part of which included a television series entitled 'Feeling Great'. The campaigns promoted better health by giving dietary advice, encouraging the habit of regular exercise and avoidance of smoking and by trying, in general, to encourage an attitude which looks upon the body as an organism which, given the right care, will give better service and a sense of well-being. Many of us I suspect pay more attention to our cars than ourselves. Lack of servicing of cars may lead to expensive repairs but they pale into insignificance compared with the human cost of unhappiness let alone the cost of treatment of illnesses which we know can be prevented by following a healthy lifestyle. I was most interested to hear that follow-up surveys have shown that the Health Education Campaigns have influenced attitudes to the

2

good. What we hope to see of course is the changed attitudes being translated into action. Getting people to change their attitudes and subsequently their action needs a sustained effort often over years. I know that the HEC are aware of this and will be maintaining their momentum.

My Department plays a part in helping people to make choices by providing information either directly through DHSS publications on health and prevention issues or by publishing the findings of an Advisory Committee on the health aspects of nutrition, the Committee on Medical Aspects of Food Policy. There have been three DHSS booklets on specific preventive issues following the issue in 1976 of 'Prevention and Health: Everybody's Business'. They were 'Reducing the Risk: Safer Pregnancy and Childbirth', 'Occupational Health Services' and 'Eating for Health'. Further booklets, one on Alcoholism and the other on Coronary Heart Disease are under preparation. You will probably be most interested in 'Eating for Health' which sets out the present state of knowledge about diet and explains the ways in which diet can assist in promoting health and in avoiding disease. This booklet has sold well and is now in its third reprint. The public response has shown that there is a demand for knowledge and information of an unbiased nature − a role that I think Government in association with independent experts can provide. There has been some criticism of 'Eating for Health' on the grounds that it was not positive enough and did not identify the foods that it is alleged have direct links with diseases. The critics overlook the fact that at the present time a greater precision of knowledge about the relationship between particular foods and health has still to be established. In addition to my Department's publications there are the published Reports of the Committee on Medical Aspects of Food Policy which over the years has considered the health aspects of various nutritional issues. One of the current issues being considered by the Committee is the nutritional aspects of bread, flour and cereal products. I hope that their Report will be published later this year.

The activities of the HEC and Government are very important in helping people to make wise health choices but what is sometimes overlooked is how much the public can also be helped by those in the health professions who are in direct contact with them. I refer of course to the doctors, nurses, health visitors and health education officers. Although the medical and nursing staff are mainly seeing people because they need treatment they are also in very good positions to advise on the simple steps that each individual can take in order to improve his health. A person who is ill is perhaps more receptive to advice about the health benefits that can be had if he stopped or reduced smoking, ate and drank sensibly and took a little exercise.

It is not an easy task to persuade the adult population of the importance of the changes in lifestyle that bring considerable benefits because many have ingrained habits of thought and actions that are difficult to change as well as a healthy cynicism about official advice. With the child population however we have fertile ground. It seems to me essential for the future health of the people of this country that our children should be made aware from their earliest school days and throughout their school life of what they can do to keep healthy, how they will gain both mentally and physically and how a sense of well-being can contribute to an enjoyment of all aspects of life. We all know from our own school days how this should not be done. Being compelled to eat beetroot, or to go for runs as a punishment is not the way to educate a child about healthy lifestyles. Yet, most children have a natural vitality and interest and respond much more to a positive approach of how to keep themselves healthy rather than a series of threats, of 'do nots' and warnings of dire consequences. Indeed, as you know, for many children to tell them not to do something often brings an opposite response to the well meaning intention. A lot is being done in the schools. The Health Education Council and the Schools Council have worked closely together on curriculum materials but there are inevitably considerable competing pressures from the conventional educational subjects. I talked earlier about the important role that health professionals play because of their person to person contacts with patients. It seems to me that teachers and all those whose work brings them into contact with children and young persons are also in a good position to spread the positive message of the maintenance of health not just in the formal manner but in an unobtrusive way during the day-to-day interaction and discussions between teachers and pupils. I was encouraged to read in the Department of Education and Science's consultative document 'A Framework for the School Curriculum', published in January 1980 that health education was one of the subjects that it was suggested schools should encompass as part of the preparation of young people for all aspects of adult life.

I have talked at some length about what is being done to help the individual to make wise choices. Much valuable work is being done but the work cannot be viewed in isolation as the individual is subject to many pressures that influence his lifestyle and condition his choices. In matters of diet, for example, most individuals understand that if you eat too much you will get fat and that obesity does have health dangers. However his palate is constantly being tempted by advertisements for foods, particularly on television and also in women's magazines. This is all part of the process of giving the consumer a choice you may say. Of course I agree that there must be a choice but it sometimes seems to me that an ever increasing part of the total range of advertised foods are taken up with the instant snack type of foods which seem to be offered increasingly not just as a snack between meals but as a substitute for the traditional meals. The snack food market has increased rapidly over recent years and I understand that projections to the mid-1980s indicate that this increase will continue. Invariably these foods have a high energy content but they do not provide a range of nutrients. My concern from the health point of view is that if these foods are taken in increasing amounts by individuals as snacks they could lead to overweight but of greater concern is what may happen if they are taken as substitutes for the traditional meals. These are important matters for the nutritional well-being of the whole population but in particular for children. Parents have a vital part to play in helping their children to choose wisely but it also seems important to me to emphasise nutrition education as part of health education at school. Let me say again in case of any misunderstanding that I am not against advertising of such foods but I would like to see the consumer wooed to a much larger extent by, for example, the producers and distributors of fresh vegetables and fruits whose products provide a wide range of the nutrients in the balanced diet.

Apart from the question of nutrients there is also the matter of cost advantages in these foods compared with snack foods on a weight for weight basis (for example fresh potatoes as compared with potato crisps). The cost advantage also applies to other basic foods such as bread, eggs and milk which make an important contribution to a healthy diet.

Why cannot the skills of advertisers be harnessed more effectively to promote the healthier foods? Why do school children prefer fizzy drinks and crisps to a well balanced school meal?

The arrangements for school meals can contribute to educating children about good nutrition. I know that it is no longer a requirement for Local Education Authorities to provide a meal at mid-day equivalent to a main meal so there will be an increase in the number of schools offering a choice of individual food items rather than a traditional meal of 'meat and two vegetables'. I hope that the foods offered will be from a wide range so that when a choice is made it will mean in most cases that a child gets the necessary range of nutrients. It would undermine a lot of the efforts in school to put over to children the health education message if they were only offered high energy/high sugar content snacks at lunch time. The new system will give children and schools a choice, and it is important that the choice is exercised responsibly.

Some snack type foods have a high sugar content and of course the misuse of sugar causes dental decay. Throughout the world the evidence of dental decay in children is related to the consumption of sugar. In 1973 a survey found that more than 60% of five-year-old children had decayed milk teeth. By school leaving age, nearly one third of the teeth on average were either decayed or filled and only 3% of school leavers had no sign of dental decay. This is indeed a shocking dental record. I agree with the Health Education Council which considers the improvement of dental health by preventive education as amongst the most important of all the various preventive issues. There is a lot of research being done to try to establish the most effective ways of bringing home to children the need for and the ways of good dental hygiene. I am glad to say that the urgency of the situation is recognised and there is increasing co-ordination between Dental Officers, the Health Education Council and the Schools Council.

Whilst on the matter of dietary habits I was interested to learn that public demand for brown and wholemeal bread and cereal products has been increasing in recent years. As you know there has been much debate about the nutritional virtues of increasing wheat cereal consumption, including bread, and this has been widely reported in the media. It is encouraging that the public has exercised its choice in this way as it shows that public discussion on nutritional and health matters can help the individual to make an informed choice.

I have talked about the effect of advertising on choice but there is also the 'expertise effect' by which I mean the passing of expert opinions, which are only opinions, into publicly accepted belief. It is my experience, as I am sure it is yours, that in conversations about foods and alleged links with diseases that certain foods will be said to be unhealthy – butter, white bread, eggs are examples. When pressed for the sources of these 'facts' the general response is to refer to expert opinion as reported in the press or on a radio or TV programme. Unfortunately for the general public who are seeking sound information as a basis from which to make a judgement, when scientific knowledge is incomplete, experts do disagree. I think that a very good illustration of the disagreement of experts and the consequent confusion of the public is the cholesterol debate which has mainly focussed on eggs and other cholesterol rich foods, and on the butter versus margarine controversy which relates to the kinds of fat in foods. I am not alone I am sure in having almost been persuaded over the past 2 years or so that butter and so-called saturated fats should be approached with caution and that certain soft margarines (polyunsaturated fats) should be looked at with approval and at the same time that eggs should be avoided because they contain cholesterol.

The truth is that the cause of heart attacks is obscure, and no foods can be said to protect people from the disease. Scientific knowledge is incomplete. Advertisers and some professional people express opinions as though they were fact. The Department of Health's scientific advisers reported in 1974 that reducing the consumption of eggs would not affect death rates from heart attacks. Similarly the same report advised that on average the UK ate too much fat and should eat less fat, but the report did not say that to replace butter by soft margarines would reduce mortality from heart attacks. It is interesting that a recent report of the American National Research Council's Food and Nutrition Board says that dietary cholesterol is not perhaps the ogre that some people here and in the USA originally thought it to be. To persuade people through health education to change their lifestyle is difficult enough but is made even more so when expert opinion one year may be overturned the following year by an opposite view just because experts go beyond the facts. The science of nutrition is advancing rapidly and much new work is being done but I think that recent experience does show the dangers of jumping to conclusions on the basis of limited research. The public want information but they would be better served if the limitations and reservations of the research findings were made clear in layman as well as expert terms.

Over the whole field of prevention and health education I suggest that we have heard the first stirring of a response to the message that an individual does have options which if exercised wisely can bring him health benefits. We must try to build on this and convince people that the body is a wonderful organism and that much can be done by the individual to keep it in good condition with consequential benefits to the whole of his mental and physical approach to life.

2
Diet and exercise; some of the issues

P. H. FENTEM

We have been privileged to hear a minister's view on the role of diet and exercise in the maintenance of good health. I wish to follow this by asking who will offer the choice and with how much vigour. Later in the day we will be told rather more about the choice itself, how it may be offered and something about the different health choices which some people are already making.

Almost two years ago Dr Joan Bassey and I prepared a statement for the Sports Council on the 'Case for Exercise' (Bassey and Fentem, 1978). It stemmed from a wish expressed by the Department of Health and Social Security that the existing evidence on the beneficial effects of exercise upon health should be collected together and evaluated. We undertook the task in the hope that we could provide an authoritative summary of the available scientific evidence on the benefits of exercise which might influence Government planning on health, exercise and recreation within the Departments of Health and Social Security, Education and Science and Environment. At least we hoped that it would stimulate debate. The preparation, publication, defence and general fate of our report has raised many interesting and challenging issues. Some of these issues are to do with the science and the medicine but others are more concerned with the factors which have affected the national and individual acceptance of our conclusions. Those who seek to influence national and individual dietary habits appear to face many of the same problems.

If there is to be a shift towards Government spending on preventive health measures then the interaction between science, medicine, Government and education assumes a new significance. It is clear that the potential for improvement in the national health is of an order greater than that now possible if we continue to concentrate on improvements in primary care. The responsibilities are correspondingly greater. The load and newness of these responsibilities may explain the present hesitancy and uncertainty which attaches to initiatives directed at better health through the national diet, sport and active recreation. It is unlikely that the immediate revenue consequences of preventive programmes will be trivial, indeed in the short term they will be considerable, but if we take care to measure these against the scale of possible benefit then the cost will appear more reasonable. Recently Lord Philip Noel-Baker speaking to an audience at the University of Loughborough took the theme 'Violence, Vandalism, Sport and Medicine' for the title of his lecture. In our own report we did not really consider social health. Lord Noel-Baker developed a cogent argument for spending £100,000,000 on sport, as a counter to the violence in society, weighing the spending of this very large sum against the possible alternative, which is an even more expensive penal system. We must hope that cost alone will not determine our willingness to take a fresh look at issues of health and in particular factors which influence the quality of life.

The promotion of health through prevention depends heavily on advice and education; words are dispensed rather than tablets and vaccines, with the general aim of changing an individual's behaviour in a manner which is intended to be generally beneficial. Provided that an intervention in national behaviour can be identified which should result in a real benefit to the health of the nation three general sets of conditions must be met:

(1) there must be agreement among the experts in the country that the message is worthwhile and necessary;
(2) the advice which is to be offered must be intelligible, practicable and safe;
(3) the changes induced should be monitored and their effectiveness assessed (Truswell, 1978).

What experience do we have of health education programmes in these areas? We have already had health campaigns with the slogans 'Feeling Great' and 'Look After Yourself', directed towards better health through exercise and a better diet. Do these programmes fulfil the three sets of conditions? We must presume that a change in national behaviour is intended, the BBC, the Health Education Council and Sports Council were involved, the DHSS was not, at least not explicitly. The impending involvement of the Open University in this aspect of health education represents a new dimension and one about which we will hear more this afternoon from Mrs Lorna Bailey.

Very real difficulties arise even at the first stage, that is *with the identification and refinement* of the changes which are beneficial. Emerging scientific facts, which are often complex and at times contradictory, have to be distilled by experts into specific clear, brief and unambiguous recommendations. Dietary recommendations directed towards preventing coronary heart disease fall under at least six major headings: concerning (a) total energy intake, (b) total fat, (c) dietary cholesterol, (d) saturated fat, (e) polyunsaturated fat, (f) the ratio of polyunsaturated to saturated fat. Shaper and Marr (1977) drew attention to the complexity of these dietary recommendations for a community seeking to postpone the manifestations of coronary heart disease. Despite continued attention from various bodies, the complexity appears to have resolved very little since 1977.

With exercise some questions have still to be resolved. The evidence supports the contention that exercise is of general benefit, because it maintains muscles, joints and the cardiovascular system in good working order. It is clear that regular physical exertion whether at work or during leisure time can produce beneficial physiological changes. Walking, for example, can have a training effect for the middle-aged or elderly person who has followed a sedentary and inactive lifestyle. As a result harder physical work can be tolerated for longer without fatigue and all daily physical tasks are accomplished more easily. The range of physical activities in which it is possible to participate safely and comfortably is extended. This will ensure that the activities of daily living are not curtailed by low physical working capacity, and that moderate physical demands can be met without undue effort. Thus an active lifestyle appears to be important for the enhancement of normal health and in the amelioration of the effects of old age and of cardiac and other chronic diseases. Dr Young will develop this further in his lecture.

Is there still an impediment to the wider acceptance of this proposition? Yes, great uncertainty regarding the dose of exercise required. In the case of the prevention of coronary heart disease there is an established association between high levels of physical activity and the low incidence of the manifestations of the disease, angina, heart attack and sudden death. Professor Morris's investigation of British middle-aged civil servants in sedentary jobs (Morris *et al.*, 1973) found that those reporting vigorous exercise during leisure time suffered a heart attack with only one-third the frequency of matched controls who were inactive. It has subsequently emerged that the death rate from heart disease is very much lower in those who reported taking vigorous exercise whilst the death rate from other causes is similar to that in those not so reporting (Chave *et al.*, 1978). In a study of dockers in San Francisco who were followed for 22 years (Paffenbarger and Hale, 1975) men classified as being in jobs requiring repeated bursts of high energy output had a death rate from coronary heart disease only half that of the men in jobs requiring a medium or low energy output. The level of work was high compared to that common in the general population. Thus there is remaining uncertainty as regards the prescription which may be required to influence the progression of heart disease. We have to say that there is an association between the postponement of coronary heart disease and high exercise levels which may be causal.

This raises questions of the level of proof required for national action and that which will satisfy a consensus of experts. The two levels may not necessarily be the same. The nature of the scientific contributions from different disciplines, for example physiologists and epidemiologists, is disparate and the level of proof acceptable to each also quite different. In the case of exercise and the incidence of heart disease a controlled experiment is unattainable. Montoye (1975) estimated the cost. It would involve comparing the fate of a group of sedentary individuals who allow themselves to be subdivided randomly into two further groups some who enter a prolonged exercise programme and some who do not change their lifestyle (a classical intervention study) say for 10 years. He estimated that 24,000 sedentary individuals would be required, 12,000 for each group. Besides the cost there are all the associated difficulties of imposing and maintaining the exercise programme. One thing which we can say is that he would experience very little difficulty in finding sufficient sedentary individuals.

AGREEMENT AMONG EXPERTS

There has been a relative scarcity of expert reports on exercise and health in Britain, though rather more on dietary fat. Several national committees have commented in positive terms on the benefits of exercise to health. The Committee on Child Health Services in 'Fit for the Future' (the Court Report), a joint working party of the Royal College of Physicians and the British Cardiac Society in 'Prevention of Coronary Heart Disease' and the House of Commons Expenditure Committee on Preventive Medicine in its first report have included comment on the benefits of exercise for health. However, they are less positive statements than we may believe could have been made.

Governments do not necessarily consider themselves bound by expert opinion. When we were collating our own report we wrote to various Government departments around the world, principally those concerned with sport, physical culture or recreation. We enquired whether the national Government concerned had adopted a positive policy towards the encouragement of active recreation and the provision of resources for it. Both Australia and Canada had taken action without demanding proof. The Australian campaign, 'Life, Be in it', was launched in 1975; it included amongst its aims that of showing that it is possible to be active without a drastic change in lifestyle. Our Canadian correspondent drew our attention to the Government document of 1974, 'A New Perspective on the Health of Canadians' which is worth quoting at length.

'Many of Canada's health problems are sufficiently pressing that action has to be taken on them even if all the scientific evidence is not in. The Chinese have an expression "Moi Sui"* which means "to touch, to feel, to grope around". It reflects a deliberate approach to innovative and creative action even when scientific certainty and predictability are in question. The scientific community, then, needs to make special efforts to resolve some of the debates on health-related questions of the environment and lifestyle. Until it does, the principle "Moi Sui" will be applied in promoting health according to the following hypotheses which now appear sufficiently valid to warrant taking positive action:

*Alternatively translated 'to search purposefully'.

1. It is better to be slim than fat.
2. The excessive use of medication is to be avoided.
3. It is better not to smoke cigarettes.
4. Exercise and fitness are better than sedentary living.

... The scientific "yes, but" is essential research, but for modifying the behaviour of the population it sometimes produces the "uncertain sound" that is all the excuse needed by many to cultivate and tolerate an environment and lifestyle that is hazardous to health.'

INTELLIGIBLE, PRACTICABLE AND SAFE ADVICE

The first response to anything new whether it is fashion, drug or therapy is scepticism. Some important details about the physiological changes which follow regular exercise have been described only as recently as 1977. There has been a reluctance to accept their significance. With regular exercise there is an immediate increase in the concentration of enzymes in the muscle cells and an increase in the density of capillaries of the muscle. Much of the improvement in cardiovascular function is secondary to these changes.

It is impracticability which often deals a mortal blow at otherwise well-founded education programmes. Dietary change whilst living in residential accommodation is not impossible of course, but it is difficult. We must accept that if a long-term change towards a more active lifestyle is desirable for all ages, then a positive and inventive approach is required by all who can be involved. I would not wish to underestimate the difficulties inherent in changing attitudes but the chances will be greatly increased if an understanding can be provided of what will actually be achieved by a change in diet or by exercise. This understanding and a sense of priority has to be conveyed by key persons in the community.

It appears that the level of knowledge among doctors, health educators, teachers of physical education and biology may prove insufficient to sustain health education programmes. Instruction in nutrition has not been prominent in the training of medical students. Doctors have been slow to accept the benefits of exercise and are probably imperfectly prepared for the management of the minor complaints, for example soft tissue injuries, which follow increased physical activity. There is a risk that professional health educators will become more concerned with their methods of communication than with the message. If the level of physical activity among school leavers and young adults is any guide physical education is not successful in encouraging a sustained enthusiasm for physical recreation. Students of biology have shown little interest in the physiology of man for some years and courses in human biology are less popular than ecology, zoology and genetics.

The media also hold a key position in these programmes. We must hope that they will accept the responsibility and rise to the occasion. They can produce that 'uncertain sound' mentioned in the Canadian document quoted earlier. They dispense enthusiasm and disquiet alternately. The results of new experiments are exciting news. It may only be weeks or a few months from the day of the last experiment to its discussion on local radio; the route through the pages of *Nature* and the *Times* is very fast. The pharmaceutical industry has long experience of the waxing and waning of enthusiasm for new drugs and treatment. Exercise bears comparison with a pharmaceutical preparation in several respects including a potential for harm as well as for benefit. The risks are associated with heavy exertion in persons unaccustomed to and unprepared for the effort, and in persons who chose to ignore warning symptoms indicating that exercise is dangerous for them at least for the time being.

Finally, a word about prejudice, one other factor which determines acceptance of 'advice' by individuals. Though the public image of exercise may well be improving it is difficult to overlook that we have striven to eliminate physical exertion from our lives and that exercise was until quite recently part of our penal system. Some can still even remember the treadmills of Victorian prisons; we are inviting the same people to exercise for pleasure and to improve their health. I know that Dr Whitehead and Professor Bender will describe similar prejudices when we consider the sense and nonsense of 'good food' in the papers which follow.

MONITORING AND THE ASSESSMENT OF EFFORT

Dr Maryon-Davies will comment on the extent to which there has been a renewed interest in exercise programmes. It appears to be significant, though not so dramatic as in North America or Scandinavia. Perhaps my greatest disappointment about the Government's response to these issues has been the absence of any apparent eagerness to observe and document the effects of this change in behaviour. Although such studies are expensive and laborious it will be quite irresponsible to face the same uncertainty in 5 years time or to fail to collect the evidence which will ensure that if the benefits do accrue the programmes are continued and expanded.

As the Canadians pointed out 'the scientific community, then, needs to make special efforts to resolve some of the debates on health-related questions of the environment and lifestyle'. We shall wait to see whether the MRC and DHSS receive encouragement from Government to fund such studies.

References

Bassey, E.J. and Fentem, P.H. (1978). The Case for Exercise. Sports Council Research Working Papers No. 8

Chave, S.P.W., Morris, J.N., Moss, S. and Semmence, A.M. (1978). Vigorous exercise in leisure time and death rate: a study of male civil servants. *J. Epid. & Community Health*, **32**, 239–243

Montoye, H.J. (1975). *Physical Activity and Health: an Epidemiological Study of an Entire Community*. Englewood Cliffs, N.J. : Prentice-Hall

Morris, J.N., Chave, S.P.W., Adam, C., Sirey, C. and Epstein, L. (1973). Vigorous exercise in leisure-time and the incidence of coronary heart disease. *Lancet*, 1, 333–339

Paffenbarger, R.S. and Hale, W.E. (1975). Work activity and coronary heart mortality. *New Eng. J. Med.*, 292, 545

Shaper, A.G. and Marr, J.W. (1977). Dietary recommendations for the community towards the postponement of coronary heart disease. *Brit. med. J.*, i, 867

Truswell, A.S. (1978). Nutrition education. *Brit. med. J.,* i, 782

3
What is good food?

R. G. WHITEHEAD

INTRODUCTION

The subject I have been asked to discuss is 'What is good food?': not, you will note, 'What is good nutrition?'. I would suggest that the two titles conjure up in your minds quite different emotional concepts. 'Good nutrition' has rather puritanical overtones, while 'Good food' encourages a sense of well-being, of *joie de vivre*. To reveal at a party that you are a nutritionist is likely to produce the same reaction as saying you are a priest or an income tax inspector – unless one makes it quite clear right at the start you are atypical of your profession and are not against fun and happiness.

I feel that these reactions are at the root of many of the problems which surround modern attempts to define 'Dietary Goals' and to provide practical guidelines on food for better living. Food is not just fodder or a source of nutrients – it is at the very core of our life styles.

Deprived of our customary food we soon become affected by a longing for it and one does not need to go overseas to see this response. It is always good advice to a young wife, when she wonders what sort of food her new husband really likes, to say it is likely to be the type of food his mother provided for him in childhood. Nutritionists in the under-developed countries have long since recognised that it is difficult to introduce new ideas which run counter to traditional tribal food patterns; we in the industrialised countries are now learning the same.

Food habits and our patterns of dietary consumption will only evolve as our society evolves. Unless the community at large genuinely believes that a new way or style of eating is going to provide something tangible in terms of happiness or well-being, it is unlikely to be widely adopted. In the industrial world, as in rural tropical societies, strange as it might seem to a group of academics, the desire for

17

health, even the fear of death makes little impact. These to a healthy man are intangible, the unlucky things always happen to the other man – and anyway, a short life but a merry one is not such a bad philosophy.

MEETING RECOMMENDED DIETARY AMOUNTS

The most elementary feature of a good diet is that it should contain all the nutrients we need. In the developing countries this is frequently very difficult to achieve but in the United Kingdom it represents little or no problem. In fact some years ago Thorn (1974) calculated, via a computer, the cheapest way of satisfying the DHSS (1969) recommended daily energy and nutrient allowances. The mixture she came up with is shown in table 3.1. Many were surprised to see All-bran appear so prominently. This was largely because it was the cheapest way of obtaining the vitamins which are routinely added to breakfast cereal products and of course it had the added advantage of providing dietary fibre, although few thought that important then. The cost of this mixture in 1972 was 12p per day for the average person. Even though the price would now have risen to 40p or more I doubt if this would be much of a hindrance to an acceptance of such a diet; even the organisers of this symposium have never tried to capitalise on this finding!

Table 3.1   Composition of least cost diet for 1972 (Thorn, 1974) to satisfy the nutrient needs of the average man

Margarine	71 g
Potatoes	111 g
Carrots	3 g
Frozen orange juice	43 g
White bread	318 g
All-bran	129 g
Total cost 12p/day	

The textbook way of achieving all the nutrients we need is of course to eat a balanced diet and figure 3.1 shows a typical way of presenting this advice (The Nutrition Information Centre, 1960). The idea is that at least once a day, and preferably at each meal, one chooses a component from every major food group. Until about 5–10 years ago this was the main feature of public nutrition education. A more modern, Swedish, way of teaching the same general principles is given in figure 3.2. Here a triangular device is used to indicate those components of the diet like milk, cereal products, and vegetables which are needed in greater quantities than other food components like meat. This diagram has taken account of what have now popularly been called Dietary Goals.

FOOD FOR THE EXPECTANT AND NURSING MOTHER

Expectant mother

Extra food needed for baby and to maintain health of mother

Drink at least 1 pt. milk daily

Nursing mother

Extra food needed to build up mother and provide milk for baby

Drink at least 1½ pts. milk daily

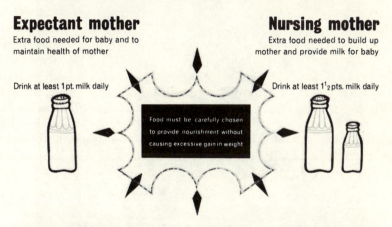

Food must be carefully chosen to provide nourishment without causing excessive gain in weight

Choose foods from each of these groups every day

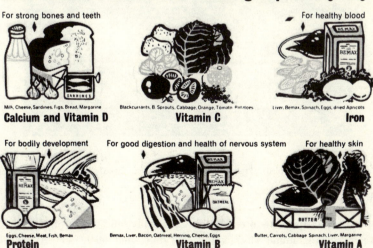

For strong bones and teeth

Milk, Cheese, Sardines, Figs, Bread, Margarine
Calcium and Vitamin D

Blackcurrants, B. Sprouts, Cabbage, Orange, Tomato, Potatoes
Vitamin C

For healthy blood

Liver, Bemax, Spinach, Eggs, dried Apricots
Iron

For bodily development

Eggs, Cheese, Meat, Fish, Bemax
Protein

For good digestion and health of nervous system

Bemax, Liver, Bacon, Oatmeal, Herring, Cheese, Eggs
Vitamin B

For healthy skin

Butter, Carrots, Cabbage Spinach, Liver, Margarine
Vitamin A

Figure 3.1 Example of nutrition education poster illustrating essential food groups

19

DIETARY GOALS

During the past few years a large number of countries have set up groups of health experts to work out just what is the best food for people to eat. I suppose

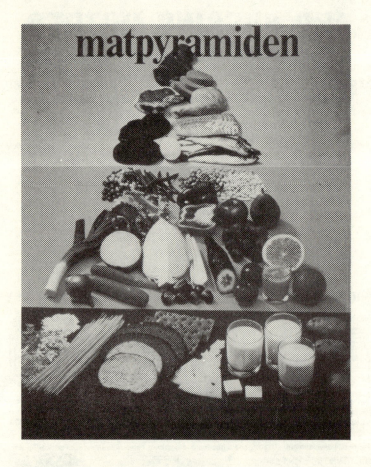

Figure 3.2 Nutritional food pyramid produced by the Swedish Nutrition Foundation

the Swedes were the first to tackle this issue really seriously through their 'Diet and Exercise Programme' (Isaksson, 1978), but what really set matters alight were the Dietary Goals for the United States produced under the chairmanship of Senator McGovern (Select Committee on Nutrition and Human Needs, 1977). Expressed in such a forthright style there was no doubt what they implied, both in terms of claims for the better standard of health which would accrue if the new style of diet were adopted, and what was expected of the farming and food industry.

Quite apart from the sociological issues referred to in my introduction, these Goals hit two main criticisms. First, there was by no means absolute scientific proof for the health claims being made, and secondly there would have been chaos in the agricultural and food world if the American public had seen the light overnight and followed Senator McGovern's lead.

I would like to think we have now reached a position where we can stand back and take a fresh look at the dietary goals issue. Table 3.2 summarises what

Table 3.2   General components of dietary recommendations produced for industrialised countries

1.	Eat rather less sugar
2.	Reduce fat intake
3.	Moderate alcohol consumption
4.	Add less table salt to food
5.	Balance energy intake with carbohydrate
6.	Eat more dietary fibre

I consider to be the common ground between the various proposals that have been made. It is worth emphasising that for *all* these recommendations we have too little scientific evidence to attempt anything more quantitative (Whitehead, 1979). Essentially these pieces of dietary advice represent those horses that the majority of nutritionists and health workers would probably back.

Whilst it is right that nutritional teachers should inform the public about their conclusions, it is important that this should be done in such a way that the public are not misled into the belief that each and every facet has been proven beyond doubt. I realise that this rather indefinite approach is out of step with present day standards of mass-media communication, but then I feel that the capacity for understanding of the average man in the street is frequently under-estimated.

THE STANDARD MAN

There is a tendency in nutritional circles to assume that all people of a given age and sex should be essentially the same and what is medically and socially desirable for the standard man is desirable for all. Thus, for example, one should deviate as little as possible from the Metropolitan Life Insurance ideal weights for height and it is tacitly assumed that it is abnormal to be otherwise and, regardless of metabolic predisposition, diet should be manipulated so that everyone would eventually fit into the same mould.

There can be no denying that obesity *per se* is also associated with a number of undesirable side effects, some of which influence morbidity, but surely we are in danger of over-simplifying issues. People clearly are different both in build and temperament. Ideally, what we should do is to think of individual dietary requirements which would enable different physiological categories of people to grow and function up to their own optimal, or chosen, way of life.

This would be something like what can be achieved in animal nutrition, but here it is possible because we can have clearer objectives. The main aim is usually to produce a carcass of a given size and composition as quickly and economically as possible. Sometimes it is function which is the predominant consideration, such as with a greyhound or racehorse. With man, however, needs are usually much more complex; rarely is there just one predominant function and the optimum level of dietary intake may well vary from function to function. For example, it may indeed produce better statistical chances for longevity if a 180 cm man weighs only 70 kg, but if that man can only maintain this weight by permanently restricting his dietary intake to 1800 kcal/d or less, a situation which would not be uncommon, this may not be compatible with an acceptable sense of well-being and general happiness. I admit well-being and happiness are rather nebulous things, but they are nonetheless real. I appreciate that by saying this I am not providing any practical advice, but I do hope it may caution against a too dictatorial approach. Life is full of compromises: the exclusive achievement of a single objective may be impracticable because of other pressures of life but this does not mean we should not seek an effective compromise.

SPECIAL NEEDS

For some people, however, one particular aim is so predominantly important that they must be prepared to discipline their dietary habits completely to this end. Obvious examples would be models or jockeys, where putting on more than the minimal amount of weight would put one out of a job.

There are also examples where theoretical gross over-weight is the desirable end. When I heard I was to give this talk I thought I would ask one of our local policemen, Geoff Capes the Olympic shot-putter, what his idea of good food was. As figure 3.3 demonstrates, Mr Capes is an extremely large man, 6' 2" and 22½ stones (185 cm and 143 kg) and ever since the age of 11 years he has had to watch his weight – but for a different reason than most! At 11 he was only of normal weight for his height. He was advised, however, as a shot-putter with potential, that if he were ever to reach international status in his chosen sport he would have to be much heavier. His target became to put on weight at the rate of 1 stone/year between 12 and 23. Much had to be muscle weight and this could only be achieved by intensive exercise, which meant that his food intake had to be exceptionally high. While he ate mainly only normal food — meat, milk, eggs, vegetables and rice pudding — he estimates he ate approximately three times as much as his brothers even, who are all taller than he. This diet was regularly supplemented with energy and protein rich drinks such as 'Complan' and 'Casilan'. This was during his weight-building days, but even now to maintain his weight he must eat twice the amount one would expect of a normal man of 6' 2" (185 cm).

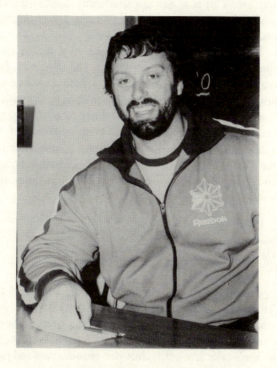

Figure 3.3 Mr Geoff Capes, Olympic shot-putter, who is 6' 2" and weighs 22½ stones

Sometimes he does 'fall to fat', such as last year when he was not fully training. He is aware of the dangers of his lifestyle, but as he said, he is a *man who lives close to nature, his nature*. He also told me that *whilst he was here on this earth he has to do what he is doing, it would be cheating himself if he did not.*

Being 8 stones (51 kg) overweight he has had difficulty in obtaining life insurance policies, but he would claim to be the fittest and strongest 22½ stone (143 kg) man. Mr Capes considers he has built himself up to a shape and size which is natural for him.

Although the example I have given perhaps represents an extreme case, he does illustrate an important basic principle. There can be no single answer to the question of what represents good nutrition. This is bound to depend on what one wants to get out of life. It is just as true to say 'we can eat to what we want to be' as 'we are what we eat'. Longevity can only be one parameter of health – life is for living too. Although it is the responsibility of a nutritionist to unravel the physiological processes that link diet to health and thus enable factual advice to be provided, it can never be his responsibility to tell people how they should live. This is a mistake that many health educationalists are now making and I feel they are unlikely to make a real impact while they adopt this approach.

Having made this point I would still emphasise that the advice summarised in table 3.2 represents good general counselling. The important proviso is that they should be adopted intelligently. Even the 'standard' person with an 'average' lifestyle should not try to impose on himself food habits with an inflexible and uncritical rigidity. There will always be times when it may be socially or personally desirable to eat definitely *immoderate* amounts of sugar, fat or alcohol, and as long as these events do not become a general habit there should be little need for worry. The human body has a flexible metabolism which can deal with a remarkable diversity of events; it is the continuous insult which tends to lead to undesirable consequences.

GOOD FOOD IN AN INTERNATIONAL PERSPECTIVE

I began this paper by suggesting that 'good nutrition' and 'good food' conjure up totally different emotional responses. I hope that what has been said will help to convince you that much of this is due to an over-reaction on the part of the public, popular educators and would-be legislators alike. It is not impossible to have one's cake and eat it, but this requires care and judgement and only the individual can decide on the optimal balance for him.

At least in countries like the United Kingdom, we are lucky. We do have the opportunity to make an informed choice. Any likely range of foods we might choose to eat could, given time, be made available in sufficient quantities. Consider the problems of many developing countries. Whatever research we nutritionists might do, whatever we may advise is largely pointless; there is usually just not the finance for most Governments and people to respond. I do not apologise for concluding with figure 3.4. For such people dietary

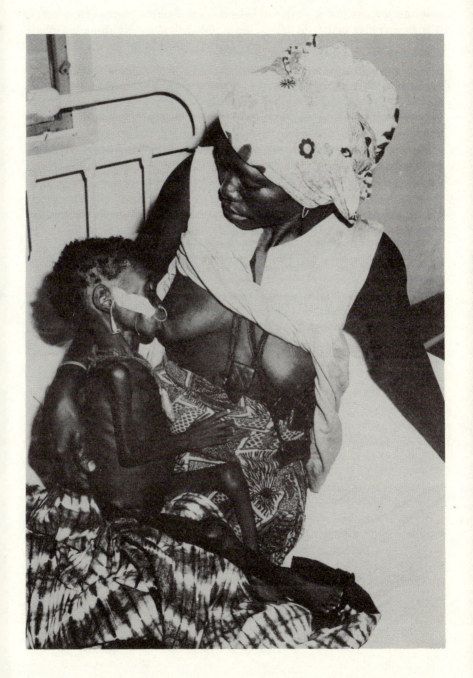

Figure 3.4 Marasmic child and nursing mother from The Gambia

problems are not just a matter of balancing one desirable fancy with another, it is an everyday matter of life or death. Good food and nutrition is a global question – we are in danger of becoming too parochial in our thinking about this subject.

References

DHSS (1969). Recommended Intakes of Nutrients for the United Kingdom. *Rep. Pub. Hlth med. Subj.*, **120**, London: HMSO

Isaksson, B. (1978). Swedish Diet and Exercise Programme. Report presented at 2nd Internat. Congr. Obesity, Washington, D.C., 1977, reproduced in *BNF Nutrition Bulletin*, **4**, 228–33

The Nutrition Information Centre Vitamins Ltd., London (1960). Food for expecting and nursing mothers

Select Committee on Nutrition and Human Needs (1977). *Dietary Goals for the United States*. Washington, D.C. : US Government Printing Office, 81-6050

Thorn, J. (1974). Low cost diets and their formulation by computer. *Nutrition, Lond.*, **28**, 31–38

Whitehead, R. G. (1979). Dietary Allowances of Energy and Nutrients. In: *Biochemistry of Nutrition* IA, 27, 281–325 (Ed. A. Neuberger and T. H. Jukes). Baltimore: University Park Press.

4
The mythology of food

A. E. BENDER

There are myths attached to every field of human experience and since food consumption is a universal pastime foods carry their fair share of such beliefs. They have done so since the earliest days when men believed that eating the heart of their enemies would give them strength, pigs' trotters would render them fleet of foot, and that powdered rhinoceros horn would render miracles of virility. It is possible that in some areas these same myths persist. For example, it is reliably reported that the Army Regulations of Malagasy forbid soldiers to eat hedgehogs since these creatures retreat backwards when approached and might confer cowardly habits on their consumers.

Since food has played so vital a role in human history we must expect an extensive mythology to be built around the subject. Esau sold his birthright for bread and a potage of lentils; it was famine in the Middle East that brought Jacob and his family to settle in Egypt, and it was famine in Ireland 4000 years later that established the New York police force. We are told that Napoleon lost the battle of Leipzig because his mind was clouded after a heavy meal of shoulder of mutton stuffed with onions, that the Indian mutiny was triggered off by the use of pig fat on the cartridges, and that the search for spices led to the establishment of the British Empire.

Some of the older myths, which may, indeed, still be believed, include the belief that toast makes the hair curl, that fish makes brains and, in certain parts of England, that a mouse sandwich will cure the cold. These have been thoroughly investigated by social nutritionists and are being superseded by newer ideas.

SPINACH

One of the best known 'facts' about food is that spinach is good for you. While a major source of this information must have been the Popeye Nutritional

School of Hollywood, the fact seems to have been well known by Victorian nannies building the bodies and aversions of their charges.

I am indebted to Professor den Hartog of Holland for tracing the possible origin of this belief. It started in 1870 when Dr E. von Wolff published food analyses showing that spinach was exceptionally rich in iron – a figure that was repeated in several textbooks until it was re-analysed by Professor Schupan in 1937. His analysis showed that the iron content of spinach was little different from that of other green vegetables and was one tenth of that originally reported. It seems possible that the fame of spinach rested on a misplaced decimal point (table 4.1).

Table 4.1

	Iron (mg/100 g)	
Boiled	spinach	4.0
	turnip tops	3.1
	leeks	2.0
Raw	parsley	8.0
	endive	2.8

In these days when processed foods are criticised it is interesting to recall that Popeye derived his powers from canned not from fresh spinach. Whether this was a hidden plot by American food manufacturers in an attempt to forestall criticisms of processed foods that were to arise a generation later has still to be determined.

In modern days we try to find the origins of ancient mythology, but many of our feasible explanations may be completely incorrect. Now that we know something of the action of penicillin some people explain why a century or two ago people ate mouldy buns as a cure for disease. It sounds credible until one finds: (1) that the strain of penicillium was wrong, and (2) that the amount present would have been quite ineffective.

So almost any beliefs about spinach can be 'explained' in the light of present knowledge. It is so rich in carotene that 100 g will provide enough vitamin A for two days, and 100% of the recommended daily amount of calcium; next to asparagus it is the richest of all vegetables as a source of vitamin E – and the myths about vitamin E itself, all quite untrue, allow almost any story about spinach to be believed.

If spinach should ever achieve a bad reputation then that can be explained by (1) its high content of oxalic acid, not only a toxin but a substance that can prevent the absorption of a range of minerals; (2) its ability to form nitrite immediately after being harvested, a substance which in turn, can combine with secondary amines from other foods and actually form detectable amounts of carcinogens (nitrosamines) in the stomach of the consumer.

In fact, on the basis of protein content per 100 g of cooked food, 5 g spinach is as rich in protein as most of the legumes (4—8 g) — renowned for being poor man's meat, meaning excellent sources of protein.

There is usually an amazingly great difference between the protein content of raw and cooked foods. For example, rice contains 6.5 g of protein per 100 g when purchased; after it has been cooked this value falls to 2.2 g — which might be looked upon by some as inefficiency in cooking. But, of course, the protein does not disappear with the cooking water, it has simply been diluted, so it is more correct to measure protein as a proportion of the total energy content — protein energy per cent. As the rice absorbs water both its energy and protein are equally diluted so that the protein content is 7.2% of the total energy when raw, and the same when cooked.

Having agreed that this is the most useful method of stating protein content let us look at the protein content of spinach, and compare it with the protein-rich legumes (table 4.2).

Now we find that spinach contains 67% of its energy as protein, cabbage contains 58%, and turnip tops as much as 98%. Legumes are, as we originally

Table 4.2

Food	Protein (g/100 g food)	Energy (kcal)	Protein (energy per cent)
Broad beans, cooked	4.1	48	34
Butter beans, cooked	7.1	95	30
Haricot, cooked	6.6	93	28
Lentils, cooked	7.6	99	31
Fresh peas	5.8	67	35
Dried peas	21.6	286	30
Chick peas, dried	20.2	320	25
Chick peas, cooked	5.3	97	22
Cabbage, boiled	1.3	9	58
Spinach, boiled	5.0	30	67
Turnip tops	2.7	11	98

suspected, rich sources of protein on that basis, ranging between 22% for cooked chick peas to 35% for fresh garden peas — but very much inferior to cabbage as a source of protein.

FRUITS AND VEGETABLES

A great deal of mythology surrounds fruits and vegetables, the starting point being the grouping together of entirely different foods.

This group includes foods that are: (1) Extremely rich sources of carotene, such as carrots – which alone provide more than 10% of the average UK intake of vitamin A – and lesser sources such as apricots, peaches, pawpaws. Others contain none – potatoes, parsnips, apples. (2) Extremely rich sources of vitamin C – West Indian cherry at 1000–3000 mg per 100 g, or the commoner black-currant at about 200 mg and cabbage and sprouts at 90 mg, while others contain insignificant amounts – cherries, damsons, grapes, and apples at 3 mg, dried dates zero, chicory 4 and celery 6 mg. (3) Good sources of dietary fibre – celeriac 4.9 g/100 g, beans 5–7, peas 12, spinach 6.3, blackberries 7.3, black-currants 8.7; others contain very little – boiled asparagus 0.8, cucumber 0.4, green peppers 0.9, pumpkin 0.5, grapes 0.3, grapefruit 0.6. (4) Low in energy content and therefore useful on a weight-reducing diet; examples are (in kcal per 100 g) – boiled marrow, mustard and cress, cucumber, lettuce, about 10, cherries, apples, boiled spring cabbage, bean sprouts between 30 and 50, but ranging up to bananas at 80, boiled plantains at 120, avocado 220, and dried figs, dates and raisins at 210–240.

Finally we have problems in doing what the botanist can do so easily, namely segregating fruits from vegetables. From the culinary aspect we include tomatoes, cucumbers and olives among the vegetables, while melons are fruits; and when it comes to stems we call them vegetables if eaten at the beginning of the meal (celery and asparagus) and fruits if eaten at the end of the meal, rhubarb. The avocado does not seem to have been classified in nutrition or cookery books.

So when the school child will not eat his spinach or cabbage or rhubarb and asks why he should, we may be forced to discuss the acid-base balance, or the specific chemical substances like hydroxyphenyl isatin in prunes that confer special properties on the food. Plantains, and other members of the Musa species contain 5-hydroxytryptamine and, when eaten in the large amounts as are eaten in Uganda, they are suspected of having an effect on the circulatory and central nervous systems. Potatoes contain solanine, peanuts and brassicas contain goitrogens, strawberries, rhubarb, spinach contain oxalic acid. So they almost all contain toxins that would not be permitted in manufactured foods. Just to confuse the issue the acid tasting fruits leave an alkaline residue in the body since the organic acid is completely oxidised leaving the sodium behind.

The calcium is said to be unavailable in spinach, chard, sorrel, parsley and beet greens, and a number – beans, broccoli, sprouts, cabbage, leeks, onions, radishes, turnips – are termed gas-formers.

Garlic lowers blood cholesterol, liquorice root has an aldosterone effect, and Durian fruit has its own Eastern mythology as a source of virility.

This great variety of foods with their differing nutritional, physiological and pharmacological functions was described by one major food manufacturer as 'unexciting plate fillers!'.

BREAD

Despite the varied and abundant diet in this country, cereals, particularly bread, continue to provide a large part of our energy and protein intake, and some of the vitamins and minerals. Two factors, however, have militated against bread — one is that it is 'fattening' and the other is that factory bread is devoid of nutrients.

This modern myth causes problems in the feeding of families since some mothers believe it to such an extent that they are chary of giving bread, or at least 'too much' bread, to their growing family.

'Fattening', of course, is an indefinable term — all food is fattening if enough is eaten. In fact no food is fattening to those individuals, the majority it seems, who burn off the surplus. Fattening cannot be measured in terms of energy density since the food may be normally eaten in small quantities — doubtless caviare has a high energy content per 100 g, and certainly parsley is one of the richest sources of nutrients per 100 g (that much would supply the entire day's recommended amount of iron, of vitamin A, 500% of the vitamin C, and a large amount of dietary fibre — but few people are likely to eat parsley regularly in such amounts). So 'fattening' might well be measured in terms of energy per quantity usually eaten. In that case many foods could be described as fattening.

As regards bread, many very peculiar descriptions have been given to white bread by a range of ill-informed persons. Those familiar with the national food survey know that even with the considerable removal of nutrients that takes place when the grain is milled to white flour, it still is capable of making a major contribution to the diet. The bread industry must certainly be aware of the problem of destroying myths.

Certain other foods have recently been victims of mythology to the detriment of sales. It is said that a well-known American manufacturer of minced beef patties had to spend some quarter of a million dollars advertising the facts of his product to counter a myth that it was made with worms. The story apparently gained considerable credence despite the fact that any fisherman or gardener would have explained that worms cost far more than beef.

A sweet on sale in the United States was said, by the very schoolboys expected to be customers, to be a cause of cancer. This story also cost a great deal to overcome.

Manufacturers are uncertain how such myths arise and may even blame their rivals. One manufacturer of a sugary drink of universal fame refused to pay good money to defend the product against the story that it dissolved the teeth but instead, threatened to sue for the usual million dollars anyone repeating the story. Without chancing a slander suit it is worth recalling that about 30 years ago when Dr Charles Hill was Minister of Food, a question was asked in the House of Commons about the acidity of a certain Cola drink and its effect on teeth. The question achieved immortal fame among chemists because pH was mentioned and defined in the House of Commons. When it was stated that the pH of the drink in question was 3.5, the question was 'what is pH?' The Minister after having received notice of the question and being briefed by experts, duly replied that it was the reciprocal of the logarithm of the hydrogen ion concentration. A subsequent letter in the *Times* stated that this was an incorrect answer, since pH was, in fact, the negative logarithm of the hydrogen ion concentration!

On similar lines is a myth dating from the First World War that raspberry jam contained wooden pips to mislead the consumer into believing that it had a high fruit content. The fact that a single raspberry per jar of jam would be much cheaper than employing skilled carpenters to fashion pips does nothing to destroy the myth – it is still believed by those who ate the jam at that time – and we still await definitive evidence from the food scientists.

SPORTS AND ATHLETICS

It is a truism to say that people believe what they want to believe, and this lies at the root of so many beliefs about what are wrongly, and often dishonestly, called health foods. Athletes of championship status need to be superior to their opponents by only the smallest fraction in order to win, so any factor that might possibly induce this improvement in performance, however small, is eagerly sought. Consequently any suggestion that a food might have a beneficial effect is listened to and adopted.

In *Nutrition Today* (Winter 1970) Dr Hanley visited the crews training for the oldest continuous sporting event in the world, the America's cup, 'to learn if any milestones in nutrition progress were being passed by them'.

The French crew had their own chef and for three months away from home drank only water bottled in France, and made their soups with Vichy, Evian and Perrier water. A French dietitian supervised the meals. The author saw jars of wheat germ and honey, and counted twenty bottles of vitamin E capsules; all butter was clarified 'because the skimmed portion is bad for the liver'. Breakfast included Rice Krispies and 'unfermented cheese'.

The Australians 'did not bother with vitamins' – presumably apart from those they consumed in their vast intake of steaks, vegetables and fruits.

The American crew relied on home cooking by a cook with no formal training.

All boats carried on board 'electrolyte replacers', namely Sports Cola, Gatorade and similar salty fruit solutions.

HEALTH FOODS

Some of the most firmly entrenched myths involve the mis-named health foods.

Whether or not whole grain, balanced B vitamins and seaweed are worth eating matters little beside the fantastic claims made for their health-giving properties. The Hunzas and Georgians, and the Bulgars, who all coincidentally live to the great age of 107, achieve this through their foods – yogurt, vegetables, honey, raw foods or whatever is being plugged at the moment. One of the ploys of health food vendors is the magical nature of certain foods. These are ones little eaten in the country where they are to be sold although they may be common elsewhere. For example yogurt was once acclaimed as the food that allowed or even stimulated the Bulgars to live to 107 until the ordinary food manufacturers made it available to all. So now the ground has to shift to 'live' yogurt. Similarly buckwheat, rarely seen in this country and so extremely 'healthy' is the food of the middle class in Canada and the United States, and of the peasant in Central Europe. Sesame seeds, watermelon seeds and other unknown foods, may be common enough elsewhere but sufficiently rare in this country to make them worth selling.

'Abundavita food supplements' are prepared from grasses grown on Hunza farms where naturally-occurring glacial silt provides them with exclusive ingredients. Such foods produce longevity, perfect health, happiness, hardihood, vigour and good eyesight – so they are at least worth trying. No price can be too high for such wonders. Their attributes are endless – they deodorise the body, clean and lubricate the intestinal tract, prevent mental depression, induce loss of weight (this may not be beneficial to all) and many, many other properties which were discussed in a suit filed in the US District Court at Cincinnati in 1960.

In China in the 6th century BC Sze Teu wrote 'sea vegetables are a delicacy for the most honoured guest' which clearly makes them worth buying today. 'Scientific studies at McGill University have shown that a substance in sea plants called alginic acid helps us to eliminate toxins and reduces our body's absorption of atomic radiation.' Similarly we can buy sea salt here at 2¼ times the price of ordinary (purified) table salt and 100 times the price of similar material used to soften tap water.

It is easy to create mythology and sales. One product – a mixture of zinc (now known to be nutritionally important), vitamin E (important since 1930), Ginseng (known to be vital for health for 5000 years) and a plant called Tumera (Latin name damiana aphrodisaica) – is labelled 'for adults only'.

Some years ago a Public Analyst stopped the sales in Hampstead of 'Elixir of Flowers Elizabethan Cheese' made from cows that had grazed on 'Elixir of Flowers'.

Hope springs eternal so many people should perhaps be described as optimists rather than gullible.

Two million Americans are said to suffer depression from chromium deficiency (treated with GTF – 'glucose tolerance factor'); one can buy in this country 'nutritional organic selenium, a deficiency of which has been widely reported to be a cause of health problems'; cider vinegar and honey 'dissolve away the fat' (no reference provided). Anyone really interested in mythology needs to visit the health food shops of the United States and Australia. The British are, relatively, a law-abiding race.

It has always been realised that a grain of truth helps a lie to gain credence – certainly one cannot then say it is completely wrong, and a rather involved explanation of just what is incorrect is not listened to for very long. So the modern approach to magical foods depends on reading the scientific literature and then producing highly scientific products. For example, it is suggested that the oxidation of fatty acids may be a factor in the aging process. If the free radicals produced can be blocked there *may* be some benefit. There is, in fact, an enzyme, dismutase, that reacts with free radicals. It is now possible to buy a product that makes you look younger and avoid old age – it goes under the name of superoxide dismutase, abbreviated to SOD!

NAUGHTY BUT NICE

The combined concepts of fattening foods and atherosclerotic foods (if such exist) have stigmatised the very act of eating. Every nutritionist hears shame-faced admissions that 'I am afraid I take two lumps' or 'I ought not really to be eating this' or 'I know cream is bad for me but I like it' and so on. We even have a very subtle television advertisement describing something as being 'naughty but nice'. These beliefs about food are becoming, if they have not already become, deeply embedded in the minds of the man and the woman in the street. It is the nutritionist, limelit by the media, who bears responsibility.

It has been said that there are no good or bad foods but only good and bad diets. We have read lengthy articles on junk foods written from the United States. Sweets, chocolates, cakes, sugary drinks, trifles, sweet biscuits and very specially condemned foods – chocolate creams and chocolate eclairs – are stigmatised. In fact the stigma is not, or should not be, with reference to those foods, but to the amounts eaten. Nor do the same strictures apply to everyone. There are many foods considered 'fattening' that almost every women in the street feels she ought not to be eating. Since, however, about two thirds of the population is *not* overweight, most people can eat such foods, in moderation, with impunity. If, as we now believe, they burn off surplus energy rather than depositing it as fat then there is, so far as we know, no harm in eating them. The harm is for those who need to, but fail to, control their energy intake. In short, there is nothing at all wrong with junk foods if you eat them in reason-able amounts. Even the anticholesterol lobby (at least until the American Medical Association accepted the evidence that dietary cholesterol has no in-fluence on blood levels) permitted 300 mg per day of that evil foodstuff.

Alcohol is a toxin but we have evidence, which we hope will not be overturned when new knowledge comes to light, that some types of alcoholic drinks are protective against coronary heart disease. Certainly alcohol in excess is lethal but in moderation is even approved of in the Bible.

At a previous Kellogg's Symposium it was shown that vitamin A is more toxic than cyanide, but that is no reason for not consuming vitamin A – in moderation.

It is not valid to draw one's nutritional information from the music hall by repeating that 'a little of what you fancy does you good'. But a little of a very wide variety of goods is necessary to ensure the intake of the whole range of required nutrients.

CONCLUSIONS

No food will confer longevity, wealth, intelligence or even beauty. That is where the human nutritionist has problems that do not face the animal nutritionist. When the human nutritionist is asked if a food is 'good' for someone, he cannot answer until the questioner states precisely the purpose – good for what? Fortunately, since we could not answer the question anyway, no one has asked for a diet that is good for anything specific, whereas the animal nutritionist is told precisely what he must provide for – more meat per unit of food, more eggs, wool or milk, or bringing the animal to market two weeks earlier. With such precise goals he can eventually achieve the required results. The human nutritionist cannot offer anything specifically good for anything, other than that vague condition – general health. So while we cannot provide such elixirs man – and woman – will continue to believe what they hope for and myths will proliferate.

5

But of course, exercise wouldn't help me!—physical conditioning for patients and normal subjects

ARCHIE YOUNG

INTRODUCTION

The increased capacity for physical work and the feeling of well-being which result from regular exercise are not the prerogative of the young and healthy. Regular exercise offers potential health benefits for large numbers of people including many with chronic disease (Grimby and Höök, 1971; and Fentem *Bassey*, 1978).

I imagine that this will come as something of a surprise to many people since popular awareness of the relationship between exercise and health is limited to the debate on whether or not regular exercise affords protection from coronary heart disease. In fact, I propose to say very little about the influence of regular vigorous exercise on mortality and morbidity due to ischaemic heart disease. Instead, I propose to describe the mechanisms whereby training reverses the effects of immobility and to illustrate why this is beneficial. I shall often refer to the place of exercise in the rehabilitation of patients. This has the advantage that the patients show exaggerated versions of the same phenomena as occur with 'normal' people. It also emphasises the essential similarity between the 'trainability' of the normal person and of the patient with a stable, physical impairment, underlining the fact that regular exercise can help far more people than one might at first expect.

Coronary heart disease

There is a considerable amount of evidence which strongly suggests that regular, vigorous exercise of an aerobic or 'endurance' nature reduces the likelihood of death from a heart attack. Recent reviews of the evidence include those by (i) the Joint Working Party of the Royal College of Physicians of London and the British Cardiac Society (1976), (ii) Froelicher (1977), (iii) Morris (1979), and

(iv) Clarke (1979). Nevertheless, it seems that the lack of exercise, considered alone, is a relatively weak risk factor for coronary heart disease and that other factors, such as obesity and smoking, are much more important. What this argument does not take into account, however, is the fact that the probable beneficial effect of exercise may well be enhanced by its various proven effects on several of the other risk factors. For example, exercise (especially in combination with diet) is helpful in weight reduction (e.g. Moody *et al.*, 1969; Editorial, 1976; Sidney *et al.*, 1977).

Despite the great weight of evidence in favour of a protective effect of exercise against coronary heart disease, it has to be admitted that the evidence is all imperfect. This is where we have to be prepared to be realistic and accept that the perfect controlled trial of exercise in the prevention of coronary heart disease (with all other potential risk factors kept constant and with a large enough number of subjects to ensure statistically significant results) will never be done. We must act on such evidence as we have. My judgement is that there is sufficient evidence in favour of a protective effect of exercise to justify advocating the adoption of a more vigorous lifestyle by most of the population.

Guaranteed benefits of exercise

Regular exercise reduces the *likelihood* of death from coronary heart disease; it in no way affords absolute protection. Merely reducing the likelihood of a disaster (which might not happen anyway) at some, unspecified time in the future is a poor way to motivate people to take more exercise. Health educators should 'sell' exercise much more positively. They should concentrate on the immediate benefits which can be guaranteed to accrue from regular vigorous exercise. These all derive from the fact that physical training reverses the physiological effects of immobility. This applies equally to patients immobilised by doctors, patients immobilised by their own reactions to their symptoms (figure 5.1), and to 'normal' people immobilised by their lifestyle.

Regular exercise of the appropriate type, can produce changes in a variety of different body systems. For example, as I shall discuss in more detail later, the capacity of the 'oxygen transport system' increases. One can also demonstrate increases in muscle strength, joint mobility, co-ordination, and the strength of bones, tendons and ligaments. These are all areas in which impairment of function is commonly associated with increasing age. Regular exercise cannot halt the march of time but it can do much to postpone disability. Even the control of maturity-onset diabetes mellitus may be simplified by an increased level of daily physical activity, so that hypoglycaemic drugs may be unnecessary.

IMMOBILITY, TRAINING AND THE PHYSIOLOGY OF THE OXYGEN TRANSPORT SYSTEM

The 'oxygen transport system' is the collective name given to all the processes

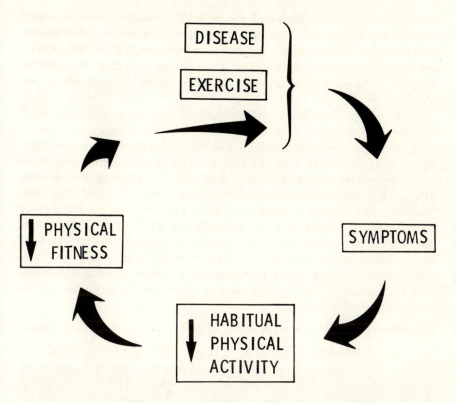

Figure 5.1 If a patient's disease is such that symptoms occur during exercise (e.g. dyspnoea in chronic bronchitis), he may be caught in a 'vicious circle'. Loss of physical fitness results in symptoms at progressively lower levels of exercise, although the fundamental physical impairment due to the disease remains unchanged. Physical training can interrupt this process

involved in the transfer of oxygen from the atmosphere, by way of the lungs and the bloodstream, to the working muscles and right down into the sub-microscopic depths of the active muscle cells — into the muscle cells' mitochondria.

A convenient method of studying the overall effectiveness of the oxygen transport system is to measure the maximal oxygen uptake ($\dot{V}O_{2\,max}$), i.e. the greatest rate at which a person can utilise atmospheric oxygen during continuous exercise. Saltin *et al.* (1968) demonstrated that 3 weeks of enforced bed rest produced a mean reduction in $\dot{V}O_{2\,max}$ of 28% in five healthy young men. In itself, the reduction in $\dot{V}O_{2\,max}$ is not particularly important for everyday life since most people rarely exercise at this intensity. However, a reduction in $\dot{V}O_{2\,max}$ means that the amount of oxygen required to perform a fixed level of submaximal work, although unchanged in absolute terms, becomes a correspondingly increased proportion of the maximum which can be transported from the atmosphere to the working muscles. The transport of the necessary amount of oxygen therefore results in a correspondingly greater disturbance of the mechanisms involved in the oxygen transport system, e.g. Saltin's subjects' heart rates during a standard exercise (approximately equivalent to walking on the level at 4½ miles per hour) rose from an average of 129 beats/min to 164 beats/min.

Saltin and his colleagues also demonstrated that the immobility-induced reduction in $\dot{V}O_{2\,max}$ could be quickly reversed by physical training. Three of his subjects recovered their previous level of aerobic (or 'cardio-respiratory') fitness in 8, 10 and 12 days and then went on to make further substantial gains with continued training. After a total of 8 weeks training their average $\dot{V}O_{2\,max}$ was 38% greater than it had been even before the period of bedrest. The other two subjects were trained athletes and they took much longer to recover their pre-bedrest levels of fitness (29 and 43 days). This illustrates a fundamental point about the effect of physical training: substantial gains in aerobic fitness can be made with only a few weeks' training and, if the pre-training level of fitness is very low (as it was in the three untrained subjects after their period of bedrest) the gains in fitness may be very rapid indeed.

Illustrative example 1 – normal middle-aged man

The 'normal' sedentary individual is, in fact, so unfit that substantial gains in $\dot{V}O_{2\,max}$ (and therefore a substantial reduction in the heart rate response to submaximal work) can be achieved with only a few weeks of light training. A 47 year old male officeworker, overweight but with no particular complaints about his health, exercised on a bicycle ergometer at a work rate of 110 W – roughly equivalent to walking at 4½ miles per hour on the level (figure 5.2). His heart rate was monitored during testing on two separate occasions, before and after 6 weeks of jogging three times a week. The intention was that he should exercise for 10 min on both occasions. On the first occasion he had to stop after only 5½ min, by which time his heart rate was 186 beats/min – probably his maximum heart rate. His heart rate was also followed during recovery after the end of exercise and after 6½ min it was still 125 beats/min. When retested six weeks later, the subject was again set to perform 10 min of continuous pedalling at 110 W. Over the first 5 min his heart rate was about 20 beats/min slower than it had been at the corresponding times in the first test. He was able to complete the 10 min of exercise comfortably and his heart rate was still only 177 beats/min at the finish. His heart rate then took only 2½ min to fall below 125 beats/min.

This illustrates that mild (but regular) physical exercise can produce a substantial increase in an individual's capacity for physical work, reducing the stress imposed on the heart by submaximal levels of activity, such as are encountered in everyday life. This is seen even more dramatically in the case of the patient

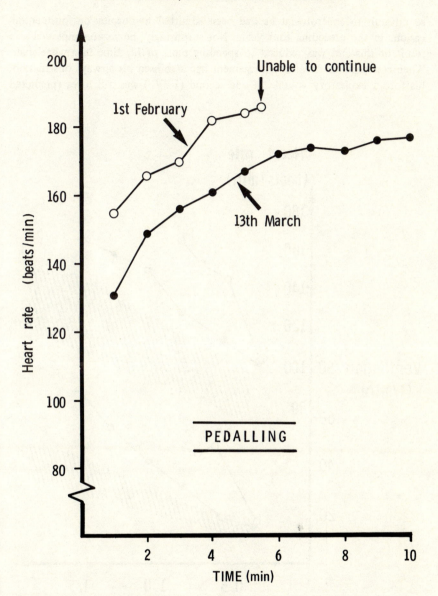

Figure 5.2 Heart rate responses of a 47 year old man to bicycle ergometer exercise at 110 W (660 kpm/min) before and after a 6 week jogging programme

whose story follows.

Illustrative example 2 – patient with chronic airways obstruction

The patient was a 48 year old man with long-standing asthma which had proved

41

so difficult to control that he had been admitted to hospital on fourteen occasions in the preceding four years. Not surprisingly, he was unemployed as a result of this and was reduced to spending most of his time in a wheelchair. When conventional medical management had stabilised his airways obstruction, his forced expiratory volume in one second (FEV_1) was 1.8 litres (predicted

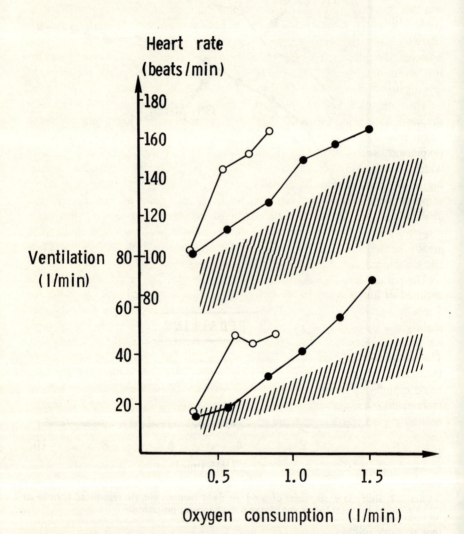

Figure 5.3 Results of progressive exercise tests performed on a bicycle ergometer before (0) and after (●) a 1 week programme of physical training. The patient was a 48 year old man with moderately severe airways obstruction (FEV_1/VC = 1.8/3.0) but disabling breathlessness on exertion. (Normal responses indicated by cross-hatching)

normal = 2.7–3.7) and his vital capacity (VC) was 3.0 litres (predicted normal = 3.4–4.6). This indicated that he now had only a moderate degree of airways obstruction. This was further supported by the fact that his total lung volume (6.0 litres) was not increased above normal and the ratio of his residual volume to total lung capacity (45%) was only slightly elevated (normal = less than 40%). There was nothing in his chest X-ray or lung scan to account for the fact that he was still very short of breath on exertion. His exercise tolerance was such that he could still only manage some 5–10 steps on the level before collapsing into the nearest chair with severe breathlessness. Now that his asthma was in remission, however, the residual, mild airways obstruction was not sufficient to account for this severe degree of breathlessness on exertion. It was decided, therefore, to investigate whether simple unfitness might explain his symptoms.

The patient performed a progressive exercise test on a bicycle ergometer with the work rate being increased by 16 W every minute. His heart rate and ventilation responses were recorded every minute and plotted against the work rate (expressed here as oxygen uptake) (figure 5.3). The maximum oxygen uptake which he was able to achieve was 0.9 ℓ/min (approximately equivalent to walking on the level at three miles per hour). The genuineness of this as a maximal effort is supported by the fact that his heart rate when he gave up was 164 beats/min — not far short of his predicted maximal heart rate. His heart rate response to this level of work and at the preceding submaximal levels of work greatly exceeded the values expected for normal men of his age. His total ventilation at each work rate was also well above normal.

The patient was then started on a training regime. The initial level of exercise required of him was extremely low — he pedalled on the bicycle ergometer for 5 min at a time with zero resistance to pedalling. The work load was increased slightly day by day and as the patient became more able to perform the exercise, his training programme also included short periods of walking on a treadmill. The use of a bicycle ergometer and a treadmill made it possible for the rate of increase in his exercise levels to be carefully controlled so that the therapist could ensure that his initial exercise load was extremely light and the subsequent increments were appropriately small. The same principles apply when a basically healthy person starts an exercise programme although it is not then necessary to use such a formalised approach. After only a week of training the patient was able to walk comfortably for half an hour on the treadmill at 2 km/h (1¼ mph), whereas his exercise tolerance a week earlier had only been some five to ten steps.

A repeat exercise test performed after the first week of training showed that he could now achieve an oxygen uptake of 1.5 ℓ/min, at a heart rate similar to that achieved at the end of the first test. At the level of exercise (oxygen uptake) which had been his maximum only a week earlier, his heart rate was only 127, a reduction of 37 beats/min. His ventilation responses were also lower than in the first test although the ventilation at his maximal work rate was higher than the maximum achieved in the first test. This confirms that his performance in the first test had not been limited by his respiratory function, since his FEV_1 and VC remained unchanged.

The beneficial effects of supervised rehabilitation exercise for patients with chronic airways obstruction, as illustrated by this patient, have been well demonstrated several times in the past (e.g. Petty *et al.*, 1969; McGavin *et al.*, 1977; Afzelius-Frisk *et al.*, 1977). Yet most doctors do not appreciate the size of the changes which can be produced and the ease with which this can be done. Similarly, I believe that doctors are insufficiently aware of the extent to which the physiological effects of immobility contribute to their patients' symptoms and disability.

Peripheral arterial insufficiency

Peripheral arterial insufficiency is another clinical area where the beneficial effects of regular exercise have been well demonstrated clinically and where some of the physiological mechanisms behind the benefit are well understood. Larsen and Lassen (1966) demonstrated that patients with intermittent claudication could double or even treble the distance which they could walk before the onset of pain, by simply following a regular training programme comprising nothing more strenuous than repeated short walks.

As reviewed in more detail elsewhere (Edwards *et al.*, 1980), endurance training results in a reduction in the muscle blood flow required to perform any given, submaximal level of work (Varnauskas *et al.*, 1970; Bergman *et al.*, 1973). This adaptation is associated with an increase in muscle capillarity (capillaries per unit muscle cross-sectional area) and, perhaps less directly, with an increase in the oxidative enzyme activity measured in needle biopsy specimens taken from the muscle (Bergman *et al.*, 1973; Andersen and Henriksson, 1977; Henriksson and Reitman, 1977).

Needle biopsy studies of the calf muscles of patients with intermittent claudication have demonstrated that oxidative enzyme activity is higher than in normal subjects (Dahllöf *et al.*, 1974; Holm *et al.*, 1975). This seems to represent an adaptive response of the muscle to its impaired blood supply so that it is better able to extract oxygen from the limited amount of blood available to it (Carlson and Pernow, 1959; Pernow and Zetterquist, 1968). Oxidative enzyme activity in the calf muscles of patients with intermittent claudication can be further increased by exercise training and the increases correlate with increases in walking distance (Dahllöf *et al.*, 1974). Physical training also further reduces the oxygen saturation of femoral venous blood during exercise in these patients (Zetterquist, 1970), confirming that the adaptation is associated with a further increase in the ability of the muscle to extract oxygen from its impaired blood supply.

It seems, therefore, that the beneficial effects of walking training in patients with intermittent claudication are probably not related to the development of an improved collateral arterial supply to the ischaemic muscles but to the normal adaptive response of muscle to endurance training. Doctors should encourage such patients to walk as much as possible (without trying to walk 'through' the pain) rather than telling them to rest their legs and so avoid discomfort.

Holm *et al.* (1975) have also argued that since successful reconstructive arterial surgery returns the elevated muscle oxidative capacity to normal levels, the benefits of such surgery should be maximised by following it with a period of physical training in order to preserve the high metabolic capacity of the leg muscles.

THE EXERCISE PRESCRIPTION

What exercise?

The type of exercise which will induce the described adaptations in the oxygen transport system will be exercise which uses large muscle groups and so requires a large proportion of the maximum oxygen uptake. In practical terms, this means running (or jogging), cycling, swimming or a programme of calisthenics such as the Canadian Air Force 5BX and XBX Systems (Royal Canadian Air Force, 1978).

For the person who is overweight or who suffers trouble from his back or from other joints, there is a lot to be said for swimming or cycling as the exercise of choice. The body weight is supported in both these activities and the weight-bearing joints are therefore spared the inevitable jarring to which they are subjected during weight-bearing exercise. For those who choose to jog, even if they are not overweight, the use of running shoes with a thick, shock-absorbing cushion under the heel is good prophylaxis against joint trouble. Similarly, wherever possible it is preferable to run on grass rather than on a hard surface.

It is not necessary to exercise at the limit of capacity (Ribisl, 1969; Pollock *et al.*, 1971 and 1972). Excessively severe training exercise will only result in a crop of aches and pains (Orava, 1978) which will effectively prevent any further training over the following week or two. Ideally, after the first few weeks of the training programme have been completed, the training exercise should be performed at approximately 60–70% of $\dot{V}O_{2max}$. This can be controlled quite accurately by monitoring the heart rate during the exercise (American College of Sports Medicine, 1975). Outside the context of a scientific experiment, however, this kind of approach is unnecessarily complicated and introspective. An equally suitable guideline for most purposes is that the exercise should be sufficiently strenuous to produce a detectable increase in respiration or, in the words of the Joint Working Party on the Prevention of Coronary Heart Disease (Royal College of Physicians of London and the British Cardiac Society) 'Getting breathless some time everyday is a good habit'.

An equivalent guide to the upper limit of exercise intensity which should be attempted by someone unaccustomed to exercise has been provided by the Sports Council ... 'Run at talking pace'. That is to say, the increase in respiration produced by the training exercise should not be so pronounced as to preclude conversation while continuing to exercise.

How much?

Ideally, the exercise should be continued for at least 10 min at a time and be repeated three times a week. We must be careful, however, that such categorical prescriptions do not discourage those who feel that they can only exercise twice, or even just once, in the week.

How hard?

As with the patient described earlier, it is essential that anyone undertaking unaccustomed exercise should start at an extremely low level and increase the work rate by small, but regular amounts. Over 30 years of age, the first two to three weeks of a jogging programme should not include any jogging. Ten to twenty minutes of deliberately brisk walking three times a week will prove quite sufficient to produce a significant training effect over that time. It will then be time to introduce short periods of jogging into the walk. The periods of jogging can then be increased until they eventually replace the walking altogether.

CARDIAC SAFETY

The risk of sudden death during exercise, although very small, must be considered. It has been well reviewed by Tunstall-Pedoe (1979), who makes the point that those who could benefit most from exercise are also those who are most at risk, e.g. the middle-aged, obese, hypertensive smoker. Nevertheless, I believe that, if the symptom-free individual adheres to the guidelines already described, there is little to be gained from the pre-exercise medical check-up advocated so widely in North America. This was also the attitude taken by the Joint Working Party of the Royal College of Physicians of London and the British Cardiac Society (1976).

It is important to remember how easy it is to be misled by the finding of an apparently abnormal exercise electrocardiogram (ECG) in a symptom-free individual (Epstein, 1979). Subsequent investigation of an apparent abnormality by techniques such as coronary arteriography is unpleasant, distressing and carries its own risks. Moreover, a normal exercise ECG is not a licence to ignore the advice to start gently, and build up gradually.

After the suppression of his cardiopathic bravado, the next most important safety measure is the education of the newcomer to exercise that the occurrence of any exercise-related symptoms should be discussed with his doctor. High on the list of such symptoms might be syncope or chest pain during exercise, and palpitations associated with shortness of breath or chest pain during exercise, or shortly afterwards. In addition, it should be stressed that it is probably unwise to exercise while suffering a viral infection, for fear of exposing an otherwise transient, subclinical myocarditis.

Those with a pre-existing medical condition or with a history of exercise-related symptoms should discuss things with their doctor before starting on an exercise programme. As I have tried to indicate, however, their discussion should usually be concerned with *how* the patient may exercise rather than *if* he should exercise.

ENSURING THAT THE EXERCISE CONTINUES

There is no point in persuading people to start to exercise if we don't ensure that they continue. This means ensuring that they want to continue.

The health benefits of exercise depend on the regular and continuing performance of the exercise. Even the highest standard of athleticism in youth does nothing to improve health later (e.g. Montoye *et al.*, 1957). It is only by continuing to be active that the benefits are obtained. It is therefore essential that people can enjoy their exercise in recreational facilities which are both adequate and convenient and that they are not put off by the minor musculo-skeletal problems which exercise can bring to the unwary.

Facilities

I believe that both Local Authorities and employers have an important role to play here — not only by the provision of sports centres and playing fields but by increasing the accessibility and convenience of much simpler facilities. As my colleague Dr Muir Gray has pointed out, it is likely that more people would take regular exercise if the provision of showers and locker facilities at their place of work made it more convenient to do so (Gray, 1979). The person who wishes to cycle to work, to run, or to play football or tennis at lunchtime or before an evening meeting rarely lacks the necessary equipment. However, he has to change in a toilet, leave his clothes on a hook and, after exercising, wash inadequately in a hand basin. The dedicated enthusiast may not be discouraged, despite being uncomfortable for the rest of the day, but the majority of people are put off by the absence of these simple facilities in their place of work. This is an area to which I think major employers should give some thought, particularly as tax relief could probably be obtained on the money spent in providing such facilities (White Paper, 1977).

Musculo-skeletal problems

Minor musculo-skeletal injuries are common during therapeutic exercise programmes (Kilböm *et al.*, 1969; Mann *et al.*, 1969; Liljedahl, 1971). Of 112 patients who started an exercise programme following myocardial infarction (and whom one would imagine would therefore be highly motivated), 40% had dropped out of the programme by the end of the first nine months (Sanne and Rydin, 1973). The high drop-out rate (which is by no means unique to this study) was due in large part to the occurrence of minor musculo-skeletal problems.

Doctors must learn to deal with these problems more sympathetically and effectively than is often the case at present. The health educator's efforts will all be wasted if achilles tendinitis in a middle-aged jogger is greeted by his general practitioner with 'It serves you right'. Similarly, if the number of participants in recreational sport is going to increase (as I hope it will) then the skills of sports medicine (dealing both with sport-related injuries and with the attitudes of the keen sportsman) must become part of the repertoire of every general practitioner and not limited to a few specialists.

SUMMARY

Regular exercise can be beneficial to health and well-being in a variety of ways. I have concentrated on the fact that it will reduce the effort required for normal, everyday activities and so greatly increase the time for which they may be continued in comfort. While universally beneficial, this may be crucial for the elderly or for patients with a chronic physical impairment.

The potential hazards of unaccustomed exercise may be minimised by the observance of a few simple rules.

In addition to 'selling' exercise, doctors and health educators must ensure that the exercise 'habit' is perpetuated. This means enlisting the help of politicians and employers to increase the convenience and availability of facilities for recreational exercise. It also means education of the public on the prevention of exercise-related musculo-skeletal problems and education of doctors on their management.

ACKNOWLEDGEMENTS

The case history described in this paper incorporates measurements made by Dr David Lipscombe while the patient was under the care of Dr Neil Pride. I am most grateful to both colleagues for their permission to incorporate the details of this case into my paper.

I also thank Dr Muir Gray for our discussions on the question of public compliance with medical advice. I have incorporated many of his remarks into the final section of this paper.

References

Afzelius-Frisk, L., Grimby, G. and Lindholm, N. (1977). Physical training in patients with asthma. *Le Poumon et le Coeur*, 33, 33
American College of Sports Medicine (1975). *Guidelines for Graded Exercise Testing and*

Exercise Prescription, Philadelphia: Lea & Febiger.

Andersen, P. and Henriksson, J. (1977). Capillary supply of the quadriceps femoris muscle of man: adaptive response to exercise. *J. Physiol., Lond.*, 270, 677

Bassey, E.J. and Fentem, P.H. (1978). *The Case for Exercise*, Sports Council Research Working Paper No. 8. London: The Sports Council

Bergman, H., Björntorp, P., Conradson, T.-B., Fahlén, M., Stenberg, J. and Varnauskas, E. (1973). Enzymatic and circulatory adjustments to physical training in middle-aged men. *Eur. J. clin. Invest.*, 3, 414

Carlson, L.A. and Pernow, B. (1959). Oxygen utilization and lactic acid formation in the legs at rest and during exercise in normal subjects and in patients with arteriosclerosis obliterans. *Acta Med. Scand.*, 164, 39

Clarke, H.H. (ed.) (1979). Update: physical activity and coronary heart disease. *Physical Fitness Research Digest*, Series 9, No. 2. Washington, D.C. : President's Council on Physical Fitness and Sports

Dahllöf, A.-G., Björntorp, P., Holm, J. and Scherstén, T. (1974). Metabolic activity of skeletal muscle in patients with peripheral arterial insufficiency: effect of physical training. *Eur. J. clin. Invest.*, 4, 9

Editorial (1976). Effect of exercise alone on obesity. *Brit. med. J.*, 1, 336

Edwards, R.H.T., Young, A. and Wiles, C.M. (1980). Needle biopsy of skeletal muscle in the diagnosis of myopathy and the clinical study of muscle function and repair. *New Engl. J. Med.*, 302, 261

Epstein, S.E. (1979). Limitations of electrocardiographic exercise testing. *New Engl. J. Med.*, 301, 264

Froelicher, V.F. (1977). Does exercise conditioning delay progression of myocardial ischaemia in coronary atherosclerotic heart disease. *Cardiovasc. Clinics*, 8, 11

Gray, J.A.M. (1979). Cycling and exercise. *Health Visitor*, 52, 519

Grimby, G. and Höök, O. (1971). Physical training of different patient groups. *Scand. J. Rehab. Med.*, 3, 15

Henriksson, J. and Reitman, J.S. (1977). Time course of changes in human skeletal muscle succinate dehydrogenase and cytochrome oxidase activities and maximal oxygen uptake with physical activity and inactivity. *Acta Physiol. Scand.*, 99, 91

Holm, J., Dahllöf, A.-G. and Scherstén, T. (1975). Metabolic activity of skeletal muscle in patients with peripheral arterial insufficiency: effect of arterial reconstructive surgery. *Scand. J. clin. Lab. Invest.*, 35, 81

Joint Working Party of the Royal College of Physicians of London and the British Cardiac Society (1976). Prevention of coronary heart disease. *J. Roy. Coll. Phys.*, 10, 213

Kilböm, Å., Hartley, L.H., Saltin, B., Bjure, J., Grimby, G. and Åstrand, I. (1969). Physical training of sedentary middle-aged and older men. I Medical evaluation. *Scand. J. clin. Lab. Invest.*, 24, 315

Larsen, O.A. and Lassen, N.A. (1966). Effect of daily muscular exercise in patients with intermittent claudication. *Lancet*, 2, 1093

Liljedahl, S.-O. (1971). Common injuries in connection with conditioning exercises. *Scand. J. Rehab. Med.*, 3, 1

Mann, G.V., Garrett, H.L., Farlie, A., Murray, H. and Billings, F.T. (1969). Exercise to prevent coronary heart disease. *Am. J. Med.*, 46, 12

McGavin, C.R., Gupta, S.P., Lloyd, E.L. and McHardy, G.J.R. (1977). Physical rehabilitation for the chronic bronchitic – results of a controlled trial of exercise in the home. *Thorax*, 32, 307

Montoye, H.J., Van Huss, W.D., Olson, H.W., Pierson, W.R. and Hudec, A.J. (1957). *The Longevity and Morbidity of College Athletes*. Michigan State University: Phi Epsilon Kappa Fraternity

Moody, D.L., Kollias, J. and Buskirk, E.R. (1969). The effect of a moderate exercise programme on body weight and skinfold thickness in overweight college women. *Med. Sci. Sport*, 1, 72

Morris, J.N. (1979). Evidence for the benefits of exercise from epidemiological studies. *Brit. J. Sports Med.*, 12, 220

Orava, S. (1978). Overexertion injuries in keep-fit athletes. *Scand. J. Rehab. Med.*, 10, 187

Pernow, B. and Zetterquist, S. (1968). Metabolic evaluation of the leg blood flow in claudicating patients with arterial obstructions at different levels. *Scand. J. clin. Lab. Invest.*, 21, 277

Petty, T.L., Nett, L.M., Finigan, M.M., Brink, G.A. and Corsello, P.R. (1969). A comprehensive care programme for chronic airway obstruction. *Ann. intern. Med.*, 70, 1109

Pollock, M.L., Broida, J., Kendrick, Z., Miller, H.S., Janeway, R. and Linnerud, A.C. (1972). Effects of training two days per week at different intensities on middle-aged men. *Med. Sci. Sports*, 4, 192

Pollock, M.L., Miller, H.S., Janeway, R., Linnerud, A.C., Robertson, B. and Valentino, R. (1971). Effects of walking on body composition and cardiovascular function of middle-aged men. *J. appl. Physiol.*, 30, 126

Ribisl, P.M. (1969). Effects of training upon maximal oxygen uptake of middle-aged men. *Int. Z. Angew. Physiol.*, 27, 154

Royal Canadian Air Force (1978). *Physical Fitness.* Harmondsworth: Penguin Books

Saltin, B., Blomqvist, G., Mitchell, J.H., Johnson, R.L., Wildenthal, K. and Chapman, C.B. (1968). Response to exercise after bedrest and training. *Circulation*, 38, Suppl. 7

Sanne, H. and Rydin, C. (1973). Feasibility of a physical training program. *Acta Med. Scand.*, Suppl. 551, 59

Sidney, K.H., Shephard, R.J. and Harrison, J.E. (1977). Endurance training and body composition of the elderly. *Am. J. clin. Nutr.*, 30, 326

Tunstall-Pedoe, D. (1979). Exercise and sudden death. *Brit. J. Sports Med.*, 12, 215

Varnauskas, E., Björntorp, P., Fahlén, M., Přerovský, I. and Stenberg, J. (1970). Effects of physical training on exercise blood flow and enzymatic activity in skeletal muscle. *Cardiovasc. Res.*, 4, 418

White Paper (1977) Prevention and Health. Command 7047, p. 44. London: Her Majesty's Stationery Office

Zetterquist, S. (1970). The effect of active training on the nutritive blood flow in exercising ischemic legs. *Scand. J. clin. Lab. Invest.*, 25, 101

6
Helping people make health choices

LORNA BAILEY

Earlier speakers have considered the information which they think it is important to pass on to people. It was originally suggested to me that I should speak to the title 'Communicating the information' or 'How do we tell people?'

Well we certainly need to think carefully about how to communicate the information — and that in itself can be a difficult task. 'How do we tell people?' sounds too directive because of the underlying connotation of 'telling people what to do'. Much health education information *is* linked with definite advice about what people should do to improve their health. Directive advice *may* be taken by people who have become accustomed to being passive about their health. Indeed some doctors may perceive totally compliant people as being particularly 'good' patients. However, it's one thing to leave your illnesses to your doctor to take care of; but, really, your health is too important to hand over control of it to someone else.

I'm making the assumption in this lecture that it should be the aim of health educators to help people to make their own decisions. We should be helping people to take care of themselves — helping them, as far as possible, to be responsible for their own health.

Even if you do think that there is nothing wrong with being directive — it's not, in fact, a particularly good technique for getting people to change their behaviour. The old adage about 'leading horses to water but not being able to make them drink' applies. Fortunately people are somewhat more amenable than horses in that, having led them to the water, you can persuade some of them to feel that perhaps they ought to have a drink. In other words, simply passing on the information, *can* change people's attitudes. They now feel they ought to make the change — but for one reason or another they often don't actually make the change. This seems to be the case with the majority of people who smoke today. They do know the damage smoking may cause. Most of those who know the dangers feel they ought to stop. However the numbers of those who manage to give up are disappointingly low. To take another example – most people who need to lose weight know they are overweight. They manage rather better than people trying to give up smoking in that many of them do manage to lose weight. But perhaps even more disappointingly – they do not know how to keep slim and soon regain the weight they lost.

It has been emphasised many times today that no health education expert should feel confident that he knows exactly what is right or best for any one particular individual. People need to be helped to make their own personal decisions about their health and about those aspects of their personal lifestyle which affect their health. They then need additional help so that they can implement the changes they have decided to make. Hence my title of 'helping people to make health choices'.

THE OPEN UNIVERSITY AND HEALTH CHOICES

I happen to have another good reason for emphasising Health Choices. And that is – that the community education section of the Open University, in which I work, has just finished producing a new course which will start this autumn called 'Health Choices'.

This course has been produced in association with the Health Education Council and the Scottish Health Education Unit. We have built into this course all that we know about how to help people make health choices. It seems appropriate to discuss the educational principles on which this course is based since these principles should apply to many other health education situations in which the three aims are also to:

1. Pass on information in an easily understood form.
2. Help improve people's decision making skills.
3. Help people build up the practical skills of planning and implementing change.

Community Education Courses

It's necessary to digress here for a moment to tell you what our course 'Health Choices' is *not* about. First of all it is not about illness but about a more positive approach to health. Secondly, it is not part of the Open University's under-graduate programme for people studying for a degree.

For the last three years the OU has also been producing short Community Education Courses which aim to help people make decisions about and cope with the problems and concerns of everyday life. These courses are presented in a popular-magazine style, with linked TV and Radio programmes and last for only eight weeks. We describe them as learner-centred and activity based. That's a typical piece of Open University jargon. In other words they are focussed on what does the student need to know rather than on what does a subject-expert want to tell them. They are also activity-based in that instead of passing on the information as just a list of facts the student is constantly helped to relate the information to his own life.

Our first course, on which I worked, was 'The First Years of Life', which deals with pregnancy and the first two years of life. By next year (1981) when we will have six Community Education Courses available we hope to have as many students on these courses as are registered on our undergraduate degree programmes.

From the start the Health Education Council has recognised that these Community Education Courses might play a part in educating people on health related topics and have supported us in our courses. They have recently agreed to finance us for another five years to produce more health related courses.

CHOOSING AND CHANGING

I'd like to get back to Health Choices and look at the process which we are trying to help our students to complete. I would hope that I have not given you the impression that I have been talking about 'them' — the people 'out there' in the general public who need help to make health choices as opposed to 'us' the health experts, in our various ways, at this symposium! If health educators adopt this 'them' and 'us' categorisation then their message will come across as patronising and directive and they will alienate their target audience. *Of course all of us here* are interested and concerned — in the true meaning of the word — about our own health. So when I talk about the process we are hoping that our students will go through I have deliberately chosen to present it in the form of the kind of questions we put to our students.

Today I am only posing the questions: our course helps people to work out their own answers to them.

This course, then, will help you to:

1. **Review your lifestyle** — so that you can decide —
   - What does being healthy mean to you?
   - What affects your physical and mental health?
   - How healthy are you physically and emotionally?
2. **Choose what you would like to change**
   - What do you need to know before you decide what to change?
   - Which changes are most important to you?
   - Which changes can you make on your own? Which ones need community action?
3. **Weigh up the pros and cons**
   - What might make it difficult for you to change?
   - Who will support you?
   - How will you make the change?

4. **Implement changes**
   - What can you do to make it easier to learn new ways?
   - How can you join in community action for change?
5. **Take stock of your changes**
   - What effect has the change had on you and your family?
   - Was it worthwhile?
   - How can you keep up your new lifestyle?
6. **Think ahead**
   - Do you want to make more personal changes?
   - Do you want to encourage group action to change things?

Well that's all a tall order. But they are the steps it's important to go through when you are taking stock of your lifestyle, and how it affects your health. We've had a shot at it and our developmental testers and our consultant subject-area experts like it. We shall be evaluating very carefully what our students think of the course when it starts this autumn (1980).

I would now like to look at three points in more detail. Choices and constraints, self-image and motivation, and the skills of self-control.

CHOICES AND CONSTRAINTS

It's all too easy to feel that life is just happening to you and there is little that you can do about it. Or that life is going past so fast that you are too busy to take time out and take stock of your lifestyle. So it is helpful to try to make people more aware of their ability – and right – to make health choices.

For example in 'Health Choices' there are quizzes and activities to help people become more aware of what being healthy means to them. How important is it to them to be physically fit? Not to be ill? To live to a ripe old age? To adapt to the difficult circumstances they live in? And what about the idea of positive health – feeling great?

There is also a quiz which asks 'How do you "see" your body?' Is it a monster that could get out of control if you don't keep careful control of it? Or is it a machine that ought to run smoothly but will need occasional servicing by a doctor? And so on.

The idea that the ordinary person will monitor – keep an eye on – their patterns of behaviour which affect their physical and mental health is a key point in this course. There is a quiz on 'You're more active than you think' which gets you to make note during the day of all the vigorous activity that's part of your daily life – and you can then decide if you need extra exercise or sport to keep you fit. 'When is it OK for you to drink?' is not a quiz about 'are you an alcoholic?' but rather focusses on the ideas that it is social and cultural pressures which often determine whether or not you will have a drink and that ordinary, reasonable people keep an eye on what they drink. This topic also suggests that you check out just how much your image of yourself as a person who drinks beer, or whisky or Cinzano or whatever, is affected by the advertisements you see.

When we come to look at the constraints on choosing and changing we soon see what is the fault in the argument that if only people knew the facts they would change their ways.

For example, suppose a person wants to make a definite change in their eating habits and so have a better balanced diet. We can provide information on what is the current opinion on what constitutes a well balanced diet. We can help the person decide if his own diet needs changing. *But* there are many other things which affect what he chooses to eat. For example what kinds of food did he learn as a child to like or dislike? Does he feel that 'people like me eat chips with most meals or plenty of bread and butter' or 'dinner isn't complete without a pudding' or even 'salads are only for rabbits'?

The availability and cost of the healthier diet he now wishes to eat also has to be considered. If he can't afford, or his local shops don't stock, much fresh fruit it's easier to settle for a tin of rice pudding. (Incidentally I once saw a diet leaflet for the old-aged pensioner which started by suggesting they cut back on the number of avocadoes they eat!)

Finally, while we are considering the constraints, there are certain problems which ought to be easily solved but which, in fact, have caused many people to give up on their new diets because they lack the skills to handle such situations as:

- their mother has cooked them the special dinner she knows to be their favourite meal.
- their husband brings them chocolates because *he* feels good when he gives them chocolate.
- the boss who feels offended if they don't take the drinks he presses on them.

SELF-ESTEEM AND MOTIVATION

What helps people feel confident they can change?

Advertising agencies — and Kellogg's advertisements are splendid examples of this — know that their success depends on helping people to identify with the way of life they portray and to think 'Yes — I'd *like* to be like that' — 'Yes I *could* be like that'.

Unfortunately it is all too easy for health educators to make people feel 'Oh dear I'm not like that', 'I know I ought to be like that' — you can almost hear the 'but' that comes next.

This second approach may reinforce the poor image people already have of themselves. In 'Health Choices' we help people look at how they may have built up a poor image of themselves. For example they may learn from their family such messages as 'everyone in our family has always been fat or well built'. Many people also learn to undermine their own self-confidence by having interior conversations such as:– 'Oh god I'll never keep this up – just one cream bun won't hurt – oh well now I've broken my diet I might as well be hung for a sheep as a lamb – there, see what a fat ugly slob I am'. It's possible to learn to talk to yourself in a more supportive way than that!

In addition there is nothing like an earlier experience of failure, perhaps because you never learnt the skills of making changes, to make you lack confidence in your ability to change. Indeed fear of being put to the test and running the risk of failure can lead to such rationalisations as deciding 'I don't believe a word of all that rubbish about smoking and lung cancer' or 'my wife prefers me to be a bit tubby'!

THE SKILLS OF SELF-CONTROL

Finally we need to help people have a better understanding of what we might call the skills of self-control. That sounds as though it might involve a stiff upper lip or gritting your teeth and bearing it! But, in fact, these skills can be learnt. Many people learn them without being aware of it as they grow up. But it can help to spell out the steps involved so that people can make more conscious and effective use of these behavioural skills.

Being able to accept the occasional failure without being demoralised and to learn how to work out how to avoid it happening again are important parts of this process.

Knowing how to change their ways if they want to goes a long way towards helping people feel 'Yes, I am the kind of person who takes care of themselves'. And this is what our course 'Health Choices' aims to help a person to do.*

*Further details of the course 'Health Choices' – and of other community education courses may be obtained from: Lorna Bailey, Community Education Section, The Open University, P.O. Box 188, Milton Keynes, MK3 6HW.

7
What should we tell people?

T. W. MEADE

'Doctor's orders' are increasingly a thing of the past. People are better informed now than they used to be and expect to take a much more active part in decisions affecting their health. To do this they need advice – which they may, however, find very confusing.

A good example of this confusion is the question of whether it is possible to prevent ischaemic heart (coronary) disease (IHD) and if so, how. Few would deny the importance of the question. But after almost a quarter of a century of debate the man in the street can be forgiven for being quite unclear about the answer. He is the victim of unresolved controversies between the experts, and of the way the lay media often present these controversies.

Infectious diseases have one necessary cause – the organism concerned. By avoiding infection with the organism through environmental measures or by effective immunisation, the individual avoids the disease. The conditions with which we are mainly concerned nowadays, however, mostly have several causes only some of which are known. These diseases can and do occur in people free of the known or suspected causes – for example, a thin, non-smoking man with a low blood cholesterol level may still develop IHD even though his chances of doing so are less than his fat, smoking counterpart with a high cholesterol level. It is consequently difficult to be very dogmatic about what measures should be recommended.

Figure 7.1 shows the individual links in the chain of events thought by many to be responsible for IHD. There are several inter-regional comparisons which strongly suggest that high dietary fat intake leads to high blood cholesterol levels (e.g. Keys, 1980). These findings, though, are based on comparisons *between* groups of men in countries or areas with contrasting IHD incidence rates. It is not generally appreciated that *within* groups with a high incidence of IHD, there is little or no correlation between the dietary fat intake and blood cholesterol

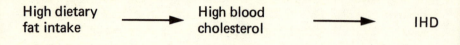

High dietary fat intake ⟶ High blood cholesterol ⟶ IHD

Figure 7.1

levels of the individuals concerned (Morris *et al.*, 1963). There may be explanations for this finding which do not preclude the dietary fat hypothesis for IHD, but the lack of positive evidence has to be acknowledged. It is also the case that with one possible and rather marginal exception (Morris *et al.*, 1977) no prospective study has shown a relationship in individuals between habitual dietary fat intake and the risk of IHD. Again, there may be technical explanations but the fact remains that this rather crucial association has not been established. Attempts to prevent IHD by restricting the intake of certain fats have been suggestive of a beneficial effect (see Joint Working Party, 1976) but are by no means conclusive. There is little doubt that where IHD is endemic, individuals with high blood cholesterol levels are at increased risk of IHD (e.g. Gordon and Kannel, 1972). But that does not mean either that all those with high cholesterol levels will succumb or that those with low levels will be immune. In summary, there probably is a causal association between dietary fat and IHD, but it may not be as strong as is often suggested.

Discussions in professional and lay media often (and rightly) emphasise the cumulative effects of several adverse risk factors. What these discussions usually fail to make clear, however, is that only a small proportion of middle-aged men have high blood pressures *and* high blood cholesterol levels *and* smoke cigarettes *and* are overweight, etc. (Epstein, 1969). Most of the total incidence of IHD occurs in those with only mildly or moderately raised levels of one or two risk factors. Preventive efforts directed towards the large number of men at only slightly increased risk consequently involve a good deal of apparently wasted effort. Whyte (1975) considered the possible implications of lowering blood cholesterol levels (by dietary and other means) from 310 mg/100 mℓ in 100 men aged 35 who are non-smokers with normal blood pressures and normal electrocardiograms. Of these men, six may avoid IHD in the next 20 years as a result of the cholesterol-lowering regime, assuming total adherence by all 100 men (an unlikely event). But eight will develop IHD in spite of complying with the regime. And the other 86 will remain free of IHD whether or not they comply. In other words, a large number of people will be put to unnecessary trouble for the benefit of a few who will avoid the disease, and some will develop the disease in spite of everything. It is true that the six cases avoided are nearly half the total of 14 new cases but it is clear that the precision of the whole undertaking leaves a good deal to be desired. It is, incidentally, important to bear in mind that diet is by no means the only determinant of the blood cholesterol level.

A large randomised controlled trial recently showed that clofibrate, a blood cholesterol lowering agent, is effective in preventing heart attacks (Co-operative trial, 1978). Unfortunately, though, it also appeared possible that clofibrate increases the risk of certain gastro-intestinal disorders, including some cancers. It certainly increases the incidence of gall-bladder disease. This illustrates two points. First, efforts to prevent one condition may increase the risk of others. Secondly, cholesterol should not be thought of only as a harmful substance, to be reduced as far as possible and at any cost. Cholesterol is an essential constituent of cell walls and it serves vital functions. The findings on cancer in the clofibrate trial were, of course, due to a drug and not to dietary intervention. But there is other evidence that low cholesterol levels may be associated with increased risks of cancer (Beaglehole *et al.*, 1980; Kark *et al.*, 1980). This evidence is not as impressive as that showing the disadvantages of raised cholesterol levels, but it should not be ignored.

The incomplete and sometimes contradictory nature of findings on diet and IHD has led to a polarisation of views on whether the public should be advised about dietary changes. Some take the view that until incontrovertible scientific evidence is available, no advice can be given. This is unrealistic. IHD is a major health problem about which the public expects and is entitled to some guidance. And much of the evidence does suggest a link between dietary fat and IHD. It may very well be that lack of dietary fibre is also a cause of IHD (Morris *et al.*, 1977). On the other hand, there are those who believe the case for the dietary fat causation of IHD is so strong that it is a basis for immediate and unequivocal action. But there is certainly no justification for implying that those who stick to dietary guidelines have nothing more to worry about — an impression that is sometimes given. In any event, the lay public is now well enough informed to know that categorical statements from scientific experts or through the media frequently over-simplify extremely complex issues, and may even be misleading. One of the reasons for this is a tendency for research workers in the diet/IHD field also to become involved in the health education controversies to which their studies may give rise. It is not easy to be objective in these circumstances.

The issues at stake have so far been illustrated by diet and its possible role in IHD. Similar considerations apply to other circumstances associated with IHD and capable of being modified by changes in lifestyle. Obesity and lack of physical exercise are two examples. In both cases, there is much to suggest that they predispose to IHD, but as with diet the evidence is not unequivocal. It is, of course, justifiable to be quite dogmatic about smoking because of its part in the causation of lung cancer. Those who do not smoke develop the disease. The strength and specificity of the association between smoking and lung cancer are such that it is in some respects unnecessary to invoke other diseases in advising people not to smoke. But the probable role of smoking in IHD (especially at younger ages), chronic bronchitis, low birth-weight and in other conditions adds to the case against the habit.

The answer to 'What should we tell people' is 'The whole truth'. This means conceding that the evidence may not all point in one direction. As far as diet and IHD are concerned, advice to the public should take a course somewhere between the extremes discussed earlier on. The DHSS report 'Diet and Coronary Heart Disease' (1974) did this well. The report acknowledged the gaps in our understanding of IHD and its causes. At the same time, it suggested fairly general dietary guidelines for good health as a whole which may also help in the prevention of IHD.

Advice on other topics should be based on the merits of the case, using the same general principles illustrated by the example of diet and IHD. Basically this means taking a balanced view of the evidence and admitting its limitations.

References

Beaglehole, R., Foulkes, M.A., Prior, I.A.M. and Eyles, E.F. (1980). Cholesterol and mortality in New Zealand Maoris. *Brit. med. J.,* I, 285–287

Co-operative trial in the primary prevention of ischaemic heart disease using clofibrate (1978). *Brit. Heart J.,* 40, 1069-1118

Department of Health and Social Security (1974). Report of the Advisory Panel of the Committee on Medical Aspects of Food Policy on Diet in Relation to Cardiovascular and Cerebrovascular Disease. *Diet and Coronary Heart Disease.* London: HMSO

Epstein, E.H. (1969). Epidemiology of coronary heart disease: risk factors and the role of thrombosis. In: *Thrombosis* (Ed. S. Sherry, K.M. Brinkhous, E. Genton and J.M. Stengle). Washington, D.C. : National Academy of Sciences

Gordon, T. and Kannel, W.B. (1972). Predisposition to atherosclerosis in the head, heart and legs. The Framingham Study. *J. Am. med. Ass.,* 221, 661–666

Joint Working Party of the Royal College of Physicians of London and the British Cardiac Society (1976). Prevention of coronary heart disease. *J. Roy. Coll. Phys.,* 10, 213–275

Kark, J.D., Smith, A.H. and Hames, C.G. (1980). The relationship of serum cholesterol to the incidence of cancer in Evans County, Georgia. *J. chron. Dis.,* 33, 311–322

Keys, A. (1980). *Seven Countries: a Multivariate Analysis of Death and Coronary Heart Disease.* Cambridge, Mass. and London: Harvard University Press

Morris, J.N. *et al.* (1963). Diet and plasma cholesterol in 99 bank men. *Brit. med. J.,* I, 571–576

Morris, J.N., Marr, J.W. and Clayton, D.G. (1977). Diet and heart: a post-script. *Brit. med. J.,* II, 1314–1407

Whyte, H.M. (1975). Potential effect on coronary-heart-disease morbidity of lowering the blood cholesterol. *Lancet,* I, 906–910

8
Are we succeeding?

DR ALAN MARYON-DAVIS

The question 'Are We Succeeding?' must surely be one of the most difficult that health educators, or at least any of us involved in providing the public with health information or advice, have to face. And yet, if health education, at whatever level, is to be truly effective rather than a series of mere shots in the dark, then some attempt has to be made to evaluate it. Such an attempt assumes particular importance when large sums of public money are being spent on mass media campaigns. After all, if lessons are to be learnt and future efforts not wasted, then we must look as objectively and critically as possible at what we are trying to do, what we are doing, and the way we are doing it.

To be more specific, let us start by analysing what we mean by 'succeeding' when it comes to educating the public about diet and exercise. Obviously, 'succeeding' means attaining some predetermined goal or goals. But what exactly are those goals? What exactly are we trying to do?

It is outside the scope of this paper to discuss the merits or demerits in terms of the content of the dietary and exercise messages that we, as health information providers, are attempting to put across to the public. But another way of analysing what we are trying to do is consider the following broad aims:

(i)   Prevent disease and death. So, in the case of a dietary and exercise programme, we might look for a decline in the prevalence of cardiovascular disease.
(ii) Produce 'healthy' changes of behaviour, e.g. taking more regular exercise; staying slim.
(iii) Encouraging 'healthy' attitudes.
(iv) Providing health-related information.
(v)   Enabling individuals to make health-related choices.

REDUCTION IN DISEASE – 'THE MEDICAL MODEL'

If health were merely the absence of disease then, ultimately, success in a particular health education programme could be measured by a reduction in the relevant mortality and morbidity indices. To use exercise as an example: if it could be assumed that regular moderately vigorous exercise has a protective effect on the heart and reduces various cardiovascular risks, then one way of measuring success of an exercise programme might be to look for a reduction in the incidence of ischaemic heart disease and deaths from that cause. This is the way doctors would measure success – the so called 'medical model'.

But if a change in death rates or morbidity rates is our yardstick then we encounter the problems of, firstly, the very long-term pathological process which we have to monitor – after all, atheroma may take decades to cause an illness or death – and also the problem of confounding variables, i.e. how can the effect of our health education programme be distinguished from other factors that may play a part, such as changes of climate, stress levels, smoking habits, antihypertensive treatments, population shifts, etc. It is true that with carefully controlled prospective studies in which defined populations are closely monitored over many years, some of these extraneous factors can be filtered out using complex statistical acrobatics. But nevertheless, any observed change in health indices associated with a health education programme will always be subject to the criticism that it is merely an association, i.e. there is no direct evidence that the change is really the result of education.

For example, over the past few years in the USA there has been a steady decline in the cardiovascular mortality rates. The rates for men rose sharply in the 1940s and 1950s then levelled out through the 1960s and in 1968 began a sustained decline, particularly marked in non-whites who showed a 29% reduction of mortality between 1968 and 1975. In women the rates are lower and the recent decline less marked but nevertheless is apparent, again especially in non-whites.

What is the explanation for this reduction in CHD death rates? Might it be, at least in part, the result of health education efforts in the USA which have been aimed at discouraging smoking, persuading people to switch from saturated to unsaturated fats in their diet and take up regular exercise such as jogging? Or might it be that heart disease or some precursor such as hypertension is being detected and treated at an earlier stage, and consequently claiming fewer victims? The fact that the most striking reduction was in non-whites at a time when the civil rights movement was beginning to bite seems to lend some credence to the latter explanation. Nevertheless Stamler (1979) has described the trends as 'probably the most dramatic and exciting findings of recent years'.

In the UK the CHD mortality trends have not yet shown such impressive changes although there are signs that some decline, particularly amongst younger men, is occurring and is more marked in Scotland. Florey *et al.* (1978) have noted an association between this decline of CHD death rate and a reduction in both cigarette tobacco consumption in men and animal fat consumption by households. They conclude:

'In spite of all the pitfalls in interpreting data such as these, the evidence is encouraging in suggesting that lethal coronary heart disease may already have passed its maximum and that its retreat could be a result of changes in lifestyle'.

REDUCTION OF RISK FACTORS

Another yardstick in the medical model for evaluation of health education programmes is to measure the effect on so called 'risk factors' present in the target population. This has certain advantages over the collection of mortality and morbidity statistics.

For one thing, the results can be apparent within a relatively short time, instead of having to wait decades for the disease process to take its toll.

Secondly, carefully defined specific risk factors are less likely to be multi-factorial compared with death and disease.

An example of this approach applied to cardiovascular disease can be seen in the interim results of the famous North Karelia project in Finland (Puska *et al.*, 1979). Finland has one of the highest CHD rates in the world, and North Karelia, a large rural area in the east of the country has the highest rates in Finland. A comprehensive community programme to reduce cardiovascular risks was carried out between 1972 and 1977. The main aims were to reduce prevalence of smoking, the serum cholesterol concentration and raised blood pressure levels in the local population. The programme consisted of information given to the public about smoking, diet, exercise, stress, etc., using newspapers, radio, leaflets, posters and groups in schools, health centres and places of work. This information was backed up by providing trained teachers and group leaders, organising services such as smoking withdrawal clinics and improving the environment by increasing no-smoking areas, making low fat and vegetable products cheaply and widely available, and providing an abundance of exercise, sports and recreational facilities.

When a sample of North Karelians exposed to this programme was compared with a matching sample from a neighbouring county not exposed, both populations showed some reduction of CHD risk factors. However, this decrease was greater amongst the North Karelians with a net reduction averaging 17% amongst men and 12% amongst women, for all three factors. The most striking reductions were of serum cholesterol and hypertension. The researchers conclude:

'As a whole, the results indicate a net reduction in the risk factors in North Karelia, which is considered to be the effect of the Programme ... We think that in so far as this project is concerned the comprehensive community-based approach and integration of the activities into the social and health-service structure of the community were particularly important factors'.

CHANGES IN BEHAVIOUR

Whilst the doctors are looking for changes in risk factors, morbidity and mortality as a measure of success, health educators in general are well satisfied if they can demonstrate a change of behaviour in the 'correct' direction as a result of their efforts.

So, returning to the example of diet and coronary heart disease, the 'correct' behaviour modification would be that of eating less sugar, less fat (particularly animal fat) and eating more fibre. Whilst with exercise, the 'correct' behaviour would be that of taking up some form of moderately vigorous physical activity involving the dynamic exercise of large muscle groups for about 20 min for at least three times a week.

These behavioural objectives were incorporated in two parallel large scale public health education campaigns recently carried out in Britain: The Health Education Council's 'Look After Yourself' campaign and the Scottish Health Education Council's 'Fit for Life' campaign.

LOOK AFTER YOURSELF!

'Look After Yourself!' was launched in January 1978 in England, Wales and Northern Ireland. It was aimed primarily at younger men in lower socio-economic groups since the epidemiological evidence suggested that this sub-population was most in need of behaviour modification and subsequent changes in health.

The campaign initially consisted of three different TV commercials (one dealing exclusively with the dietary messages; one with exercise; and the third with diet, exercise and also smoking); full-page press adverts along the same lines, placed in the 'popular' national dailies with eye-catching headlines designed to catch the attention of the primary target group (e.g. 'you'll enjoy sex more with a pair of plimsolls' (figure 8.1) and 'is your body coming between you and the opposite sex?'); and a 'Look After Yourself!' pack, which the public could receive free of charge by sending a coupon clipped from the press adverts. The pack contained a comprehensive booklet on diet and exercise, a wall chart of home exercises, a bathroom sticker showing desirable weights for height, a bookmark and a button-badge. The advertising was run during spring 1978, summer 1979 and summer 1980.

But the 'Look After Yourself!' campaign comprised and indeed continues to comprise, more than mere advertising. It was accompanied by enormous media interest, with extensive coverage and support in newspaper and magazine features and TV and radio programmes, nationally and locally. All this 'spin-off'

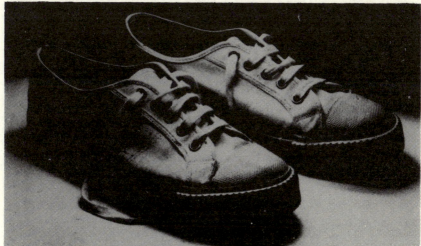

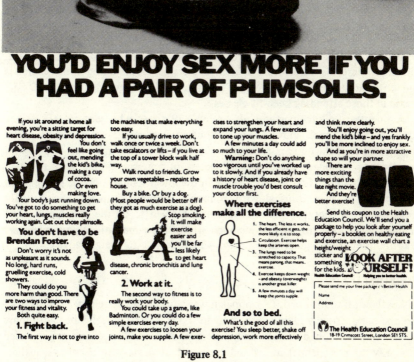

Figure 8.1

coverage led to a 'bandwagon' effect on which many commercial interests were eager to climb. Thus the 'Look After Yourself' campaign received free exposure in sports equipment shops, greengrocer's shops and on the packets of high-fibre breakfast cereals.

The campaign has become an ongoing health education programme, with 'Look After Yourself!' evening classes being developed nationally and 'Look

After Yourself!' clubs and activities springing up throughout the country, many of them fostered by local health education units.

To what extent has the 'Look After Yourself!' experiment been successful?

Market research conducted before and at various stages after the launch of the campaign has demonstrated that it was remarkably successful according to some parameters and less so according to others. For instance, in terms of 'market penetration' (i.e. the extent to which awareness of the campaign and its broad messages was achieved) its success was way beyond that envisaged by the Health Education Council. In the first two years of the campaign over two million requests for a pack were received; equivalent to one for every 25 members of the general population, or one for every ten households, or one for every six members of the primary target population (males 15–45).

Testing of the knowledge and attitudes of samples of the general population showed some favourable changes over the first two years, including a 20% increase in awareness of the importance of diet in relation to health and a 9% increase in awareness of the importance of exercise in that respect. Reported behaviour changes in the samples of the general population were less evident, but slight increases were found in the numbers of people doing home exercises and outdoor sports, a 50% increase in those cycling regularly and an 80% increase in those attending keep-fit classes.

A one-year follow-up study of a sample of those who sent for the 'Look After Yourself!' pack showed that although the adverts were aimed primarily at men, most of the coupon redeemers (56%) were women and most (66%) were married. As intended, there was an excess of younger people; and although there was a slight deficit amongst those in the lower socio-economic groups, this was much less than is usual with coupon-redeeming campaigns. So, broadly speaking, the archetypal coupon-redeemers seemed to be the younger married middle-classes. One year after the launch 30% of the sample of coupon-redeemers said that they took regular exercise and 43% followed the dietary advice.

FIT FOR LIFE

In Scotland, the 'Fit For Life' campaign was launched in March 1978, with exercise messages virtually identical to those in 'Look After Yourself!' but with more of an emphasis on a simple daily exercise routine. The campaign appealed primarily to non-manual males and consisted of press advertisements, leaflets and posters augmented by extensive TV and radio coverage of the activities and personalities involved. The public were invited to send for a pocket-sized plastic cased information pack at a charge of £1.

After one year, a total of 16,000 people had bought the packs; equivalent to about 1 in 15 of non-manual males aged 30–60, a remarkably successful response for a charged item. An analysis of a sample of purchasers showed the male/female ratio was 2:1, 79% were aged over 30 and 70% were in the non-manual classes.

The main reason cited for sending for the pack was to get fit using the exercises (51% of the men, 42% of the women) rather than to lose weight or to achieve some other purpose. Follow-up studies showed that whilst about 75% took up the exercises initially the proportion had slipped back to just under half after one year. Of those, 62% were still exercising at least three times a week. Activities other than the exercises were stimulated in 29% of the pack-purchasers, the most popular being swimming, jogging, walking and badminton.

FREEDOM TO CHOOSE

Whilst an increase in health-related knowledge and 'correct' changes of attitudes and behaviour are the major aims to health education, the primary aim is to provide individuals with the freedom to make their own health choices. Of course this entails the successful transmission of health information and the encouragement of healthy attitudes, but it means a lot more besides. In particular it means that, in order for individuals to have full freedom to choose, some aspects of their society and culture may have to be changed. For example, there is little point in encouraging people to eat more fresh fruit and vegetables if such commodities are in short supply or highly priced. Similarly, it would be unreasonable to expect the majority of British housewives to buy wholemeal bread or lean meat when these foods are not as cheap as their less 'healthy' counterparts. (Nevertheless, in the case of wholemeal bread for example, there are signs of a steady increase in consumption, more marked in the past two years. See table 8.1). Again, without adequate sports facilities, inner-city dwellers are unlikely

Table 8.1 Household Bread Consumption in the UK*
(oz. per person per week)

Type of bread	Yearly averages					
	1974	1975	1976	1977	1978	1979
White	28.24	28.68	26.43	25.80	25.06	23.10
Brown, wholewheat and wholemeal	2.64	3.30	3.60	3.70	3.84	4.86

* Source: National Food Survey.

to significantly increase their participation in physical recreation. So inherent in the business of educating individuals to have the ability to make health choices should be an attempt to educate community planners and policymakers, in Government and in industry, to make such freedom of choice as real as possible.

References

Florey, C du V., Melia, R.J.W. and Darby, S.C. (1978). Changing mortality for ischaemic heart disease in Great Britain 1968–76. *Brit. med. J.,* **1**, 635–637

Puska, P. *et al.* (1979). Changes in coronary risks factors during comprehensive five-year community programme to control cardio-vascular diseases. *Brit. med. J.,* **2**, 1173

Stamler, J. (1979). In: *Nutrition, Lipids and Coronary Heart Disease,* p.25 (Ed. R.I. Levy, B.M. Rifkind, B. Dennis and N.D. Ernst). New York: Raven Press

9
Question and answer session

Q. There's a recent paper in the British Medical Journal on marathon runners in South Africa who had been training most of their lives. These four men all died in their 40s because of coronaries and a post mortem revealed their coronary vessel walls were thickened with atheroma. Secondly, I have also seen comments in the medical press that due to the increased participation in squash we are seeing an epidemic of deaths of so-called fit men in their 20s, 30s and 40s on the squash courts. Perhaps you would like to comment on this observation.

A. Professor Fentem

I visited South Africa recently and discussed the facts with Dr Noakes who assembled much of the information about marathon running in South Africa. The majority of people who died during marathon running had experienced symptoms caused by complications of coronary heart disease in the weeks immediately preceding the run during which they died. Of course, this is one of the problems of exercise therapy. It produces considerable physiological stress and if that stress has not been increased gradually there is a risk. This is a risk often encountered in medicine when any treatment is not undertaken at the prescribed level.

As far as deaths from squash are concerned I think that in many instances when clinical histories have been taken these victims also prove to have experienced symptoms beforehand. We are talking about very high levels of exertion on a squash court possibly associated with very high levels of competition and excitement. It is a great pity to judge the benefits of exercise against the relatively small number of deaths which have occurred but clearly it has to be considered very seriously. There is a significant risk to the people who take exercise after illness without returning to it more slowly. Exercise is an effective stress, a very severe stress for the body and therefore of course it has benefits for good as well as a potential for harm.

Q. Would Sir George care to comment on two contradictions arising out of his talk. The first is between his Government's policy which directly or indirectly is causing a decrease in consumption of balanced school meals and increasing the influence of snack food advertising and his own expressed concern for the consumption of sugar and fat. The second is the contradiction between the Department of Health and Social Security policy designed to promote healthy diets and that of the Ministry of Agriculture Food and Fisheries which is promoting the expansion of the snack food industry.

A. Sir George Young

On the first, of course, children have always been able to opt out of school meals. Under the new system the meals being offered by the school are different and in many cases they are actually healthier, and I speak from experience as a parent; the new system is more flexible and it gives the schools and children an opportunity for exercising choice. School meals actually aren't the responsibility of the Department of Health and Social Security, they are the responsibility of Department of Education and Science, which is well aware of the importance of school meals as part of a child's balanced diet and sees opportunities in the new system for getting the children to accept greater responsibility for their own diet; all of which is consistent with what I was saying and not inconsistent.

On the second one, the alleged conflict between MAFF policies and DHSS policies was highlighted by a document put out by the University of Reading a few months ago which I did read and found to exaggerate the problem. I discussed this with my colleagues at MAFF and I am now satisfied that when MAFF makes policies on food and provides assistance to farmers it does take into account the nutritional issues for which DHSS are responsible. There is a good liaison and working relationship at ministerial level and official level between the two departments so I cannot accept the criticism.

Q. Mine is a comment rather than a question. My husband and I have seen how valuable physical activity can be even when the individual concerned is disabled. My husband has had arthritis from quite a young age. Although our general practitioner advised us that there was no cure, a consultant suggested that exercise could be helpful. We followed this advice and my husband is now able to cycle and finds this helpful.

A. Professor Fentem

I think that it is very clear that active rehabilitation needs to be more seriously considered in treatment that is offered to individual patients. Physiotherapists in particular have become aware in the last two years that they do have a community role to play though it will be a little time before the full impact is felt in the community.

Q. I have been trying to get information about good nutrition across to both university students and children in comprehensive schools. From my experience school is a very good place in which to provide information for children if they are to be able to make relevant choices regarding well balanced diets. I taught biology, this was the only subject within which one could get the information across. It is the training of teachers which forms the biggest barrier. If children are to make sensible choices of the food which they take at school meals, then remember that teachers are not trained to help them with their choices. How are we going to train teachers to get the information across? Professor Fentem talked about children being interested in conservation and environmental studies. I found that they were also very interested in learning about themselves and wanted to know how they could feel good, and how their bodies worked. I think if it is put across properly the information would be taken in and perhaps acted upon.

A. Sir George Young

Perhaps I could deal quickly with the first bit. If, as proposed in the consultation document put up by the DES, health education becomes part of the curriculum, course teachers will have to be trained on how to teach it. I do not think there is any problem in giving teachers the information — health education officers have that information already, it is a question of broadening it, which is primarily a question for the DES. What I will do, is pass on your comments to the Ministers there, so that your comment is noted and if we do go down that particular path teachers are prepared and qualified to teach health education.

Professor Fentem

Could I perhaps just comment on Sir George's reply? It does require positive action because in many schools the responsibility for health education is in the hands of the community nurse. There are obvious advantages in both methods of providing information and instruction. I think children are disappointed if this information does not come from their teacher and that their teacher is apparently ignorant of the topic. On the question of the place in the curriculum of this subject matter, I agree with you when you say that biology can be exciting if taught well. The problem of course is back to your comments on nutrition. I'm not too sure that there are enough people around who know how to teach it well and make it exciting.

Q. I would like to welcome Sir George's comments on the relationship between sucrose and dental decay. This is an area where there is a general agreement between experts of the British Dental Association. This consensus might best be translated into action not by just telling children to refrain from eating sweets but by educating them on the consequence of what happens when they do. For instance it's not generally known that it is better to brush your teeth before consuming sucrose because a couple of minutes after you do the acid production on your tooth surface starts to erode away the enamel and so I think this is an area where education can produce change in behaviour.

A. Sir George Young

I wouldn't dissent from that at all.

Q. Sir George, what about bicycle tracks? the increasing army of bicycles makes me terrified to take the car out. What is being done about it?

A. Sir George Young

A question, I think, that no Minister could have anticipated at a conference on fitness. Briefly, the provision of bicycle tracks is the responsibility of local authorities rather than Government. Where this is a Government responsibility, for example, in the Royal Parks, initiatives have been taken. More positively there is money available for innovative schemes by local authorities to encourage the use of the bicycle. Unfortunately the criteria have been drawn so tightly that no one has actually qualified! I have talked to the Minister responsible and he has agreed to relax the criteria so that virtually any scheme put forward by local authorities which is imaginative will qualify for the grant. I hope that local authorities who have got schemes but have been held back by the cost of implementing them will now apply to the Ministry of Transport for a grant so that we can get some more positive schemes going. The real problem of course is in the big cities where the importance of segregating cyclists is certainly higher but where the problem of making that provision is equally difficult because the existing network of roads makes it that much more difficult to find tracks for cyclists. But again I will talk to the Minister of Transport about this and I can assure you that behind the scenes many of us are active in this field.

Q. I would like to ask Dr Whitehead to say briefly in what respect we might alter our imports of basic food stuffs from Third World Countries, including animal food stuffs, to improve their economies?

A. Dr Whitehead

This is the question which lies at the nub of the dilemma. One of the conformances in DHSS's 'Eating for Health' is something like this and I apologise to the DHSS if I get it wrong. 'It would do people no harm to eat rather less meat'. Now many people have asked why on earth did it say that? I think it is because one of the ways in which we could help is that if we didn't have intensive meat production, and if we didn't use intensive cereal crops for that purpose then we wouldn't inflate the price of these crops in the world and thus make available cereal crops which could be eaten by human beings. That is a glib answer. I am the wrong person to ask a question like this. What is important is that economists and people who are responsible, do take the problems of the Third World into account when they are working out their own food policies. The Norwegians did think of this, but there is no sign in the American Dietary Goals that the developing world exists. What I really mean is we are becoming too parochial, too selfish, too narrow thinking and it will be our downfall if we don't do something about these problems.

A. Professor Bender

Could I add a general point? A lot of food is grown for selling rather than eating. It is very difficult to persuade people in developing countries to grow more food to eat themselves. It is much easier to give them a job in a cigarette factory and with the money they earn they will then ask somebody else to grow food for them. That succeeds. People tend to grow the food they can sell, and what is left over they eat, rather than looking at it in the reverse way round.

Q. I was interested in the papers we just heard, but I was also interested that there was very little mention of vested interest, except for the health food industry, and I am associated with that. I am thinking of things like plastic white bread and sugar produced by big companies as well as the more famous EEC mountains. When we talk about vested interest it raises considerations about what is produced and why it is produced. It's the companies that determine what is available, where it is available, at what price and what information is made available. We can have some influence on lack of information but not very much. I think the biggest myth of all is that the consumer has a totally free choice. It is personal preference and individual taste we should be looking at, because they have changed, largely as a result of technical and financial changes in the food industry.

A. Professor Bender

I could put up a good argument to support all of that and an equally good argument to say that it was completely untrue. You talk about information. The information is laid down by us, that is to say the people, the Government, the civil servants and the scientific committees. We tell the manufacturers what they must put on the labels and this is developing all the time. You may have seen the recent reports on labelling but the manufacturer tells us what he has to tell us. This business about vested interests, about white bread and about plastic bread, there is no profit to be made in making it white or brown. If you want brown bread go out and buy it. There are 92 types of bread available in London anyway and 75% of the people like this so-called plastic bread. So who are we to say you should not be eating this, you should like wholemeal bread and, if you don't, you must cultivate a taste for something which is usually rather hard, dense and unpleasant.

Q. If we are to make a choice, then what are we to believe? You say it doesn't really matter about bread and profit but surely it is more profitable to make white bread because the manufacturers can sell us the wheatgerm and use the extra for animal fodder. Isn't it said that white flour keeps much longer than brown flour therefore it is more profitable? And again with yogurt you said you didn't know the difference between live and commercial. I was under the impression that live yogurt contained the live bacilli and that these were good for the body. What are we to believe?

A. Professor Bender

Yogurt is not made with chemical starters. Yogurt is made from bacteria of two different types, clotting and acidic forming, but in most of the commercial yoghurts it is pasteurised so they are killed. There is no difference whatever in live yoghurt because the bacteria are destroyed very rapidly and it is very difficult to alter the intestinal flora. And even if you do, what benefit is there in altering intestinal flora?

The bread – when people say it is profitable I say, 'Well, where has the money gone?' Look at the bread industry and you find that the profit is something like 3–4% of the turnover compared to cosmetics which is in fact about 20%. If you talk to the bread people they say it is just the same one can make it brown if you wish, one can make it white if you wish. We, as consumers, are the ones who say we want the white because it keeps better. Most people are saying I like tasteless bread on which I can put something. It gives me the taste I like. It's no good nutritionists saying you ought not to be liking that. If that's what people want they do have choice. Almost every shop in the country has brown types of bread next to white types of bread. Half per cent of the total manufacture of bread is wholemeal; about 15% is brown and the rest is white so it's what people want. What is wrong with that? It should be clearly labelled so people know precisely what kind of bread they are getting.

When it comes to making decisions there is so much controversy and so much opinion that it is almost impossible to reach a conclusion. We cannot make any absolute statements; we cannot guarantee anything and when it comes to facts I'm afraid that there are a million and a half facts and the difficulty is how do you assemble them all under one heading? All we can do is become better and better informed so that we can answer the question to the best of our ability as impartial scientists.

A. Dr Whitehead

When the profit concept comes up in academic groups like this we have got to be very careful not to be too toffee-nosed about profit. I am dependent, as a medical research council scientist, on the profitability of industry.

The biggest attractions of white bread are it is light, it keeps well and it doesn't have to be bought every day. The technologies are there to do exactly the same with wholemeal breads. Whether or not such breads ultimately will become accepted by the general population only sales will tell.

Q. To make white bread is cheaper in the UK than the wholemeal bread whereas in South Africa they sell white or wholemeal bread and the wholemeal was cheaper because it had not been tampered with. To me the natural things that haven't been improved should be cheaper.

A. Dr Whitehead

It's not always the case, the more you streamline production of a product the cheaper it tends to be.

A. Professor Bender

The health foods that I was criticising are free from added colour and so forth but made in such small quantities that they have to cost more.

Q. Professor Bender really can't be allowed to get away with this. The main reason that white bread is so widely consumed is because of the capital investment the bread industry has put into producing it. This is shown by the fact that the only type of bread which is widely advertised is white sliced loaves. I don't really think the consumer's power in any way approaches the power of the producers.

A. Professor Bender

I bet more money is spent in advertising Hovis than white bread. Every survey I have seen asking the public which bread they prefer overwhelmingly says white bread. If this is what people like this is what they get; the manufacturer makes it on a big scale and that is why the price is cheaper. Its not being foisted on people if they are saying they like it.

A. Dr Whitehead

One of the things about wholewheat bread is it is not as convenient for most people to use as white bread and I would like to see us tackling this in a positive way making certain that wholewheat bread is as convenient as white bread is to use.

Q. The problem is that we ought to look at where health is suffering; a lot more research needs doing.

A. Dr Whitehead

I agree. I'm concerned about the inclination of academics such as ourselves to knock profit.

Q. Mine is an ethical question. We have heard a lot about glycogen loading which is a feature of the dietary preparation for competition among top level athletes. We have also heard about blood doping which is a much frowned upon illegal method of increasing physical performance. We are in a grey area, when we talk about diet and preparation for competition. Where do we draw the line when we introduce artificial methods like glycogen loading for increasing athletic performance?

A. Professor Bender

Add to that one, would you let athletes take caffeine or a cup of tea?
At a meeting where athletes were discussing their diet with nutritionists a few years ago one of the speakers was the coach/dietitian/nutritionist to the East German Olympic team. Of course they won all the gold metals, so he must have been right! I asked him whether he had tried this glycogen bounce back and he said that at that stage of their training he wouldn't dare interfere with their diet as the moment he did anything they would just go to pieces.

A. Dr Whitehead

The major criterion to date is whether it is harmful or not. Clearly there are recognisable risks with blood doping but not, as far as I am aware, with glycogen depletion.

Q. I have a comment on Dr Whitehead's definition of overweight. It is very difficult to draw a parallel between a highly motivated athlete who has a much greater body muscle mass and the excessive fat of the average consumer. Would you like to comment on that?

A. Dr Whitehead

This is absolutely true. Your question indicates that for most people being overweight is in fact equal to being fat, I used Geoff Capes to get over a principle rather than to put him up as a standard.

Q. Another area of mythology that needs more research is the use of herbs and whether or not (a) there is any research currently being done on herbs and (b) doctors are being told of useful herbs that could be used instead of drugs?

A. Professor Bender

Very complex because a lot of herbs are highly toxic. The practical problem is what would you have said if somebody had told you to eat the bark of a tree to cure malaria? Yet now we accept quinine. In any 100 daft ideas there might be one good one. The answer is that we don't know but the health food manufacturers who say this herb is good and then turn round and say you prove if I'm right or wrong are really trying to get advantage both ways. If they claim it is good it is up to them to prove it.

A. Professor Fentem

Around the world there are departments of Natural Product Pharmacology. There is one in Nigeria. This is one of the areas which has been seen as a natural area into which they should put research funds. There are also in this country two departments of pharmacy which have natural product sections.

A. Dr Whitehead

The issue you raise is important because this speculative research will not be done in the future because of shortage of funds. We have to accept that most research will be short term.

Q. A lot of speakers emphasised free choice and yet demonstrated that free choice is nothing to do with the way we eat. My question is directed to Professor Bender. You demonstrated that mythology of food has a very strong hold on us which implies there is a social aspect to eating which, although implicit in quite a lot of the papers, doesn't really seem to have figured in research very much. It would be valuable to turn the problem upside down. Rather than ask what are we to believe in the face of evidence from all scientific research, should not nutritionists try to understand why it is that people, in the face of evidence, still choose food more because of the way they live, which is hardly on an individual basis? Therefore perhaps the question ought to be why it is that people adopt the kind of lifestyles that they do and how, as nutritionists, can we make headway within the social boundaries?

A. Professor Bender

What you have just done is define social nutrition. It is a very large area and by my definition it is of equal importance to the biochemical approach. It was invented at Queen Elizabeth College 25 years ago by Professor Yudkin and now there are volumes as it covers almost every field of human interest whether it is religion; mother's cooking; price; free choice; sociology and anthropology. Research is going on but when one sees the size of the problem there is a great deal more to be done. It is really nutrition education because it is no good trying to tell people to do something against their normal habits. We had what was a very sad meeting about a month ago between nutritionists and dental health educators. It came about because Dr Philip James of the Dunn Nutritional Laboratories had seen a leaflet published not long ago by the dental health people listing snacks which were bad for your teeth and good snacks. The good snacks included salted peanuts and crisps and he said 'you know nutritionists are saying "don't eat so much salt" and here you are telling people to eat salt'. It turned out the dental health people have been saying for years, 'for the sake of your teeth do not eat between meals'. Nobody takes any notice. But, of course, nobody does because it is completely contrary to social life. It's no good saying to people who believe that sugar is necessary for strength, 'you must stop eating sugar', one has to go far more deeply into it.

Q. We have had little discussion about the implications of stress and wonder if you would care to put a priority on stress versus dietary considerations in relation to the incidence and causation of coronary heart disease.

A. Dr Meade

It is almost impossible to measure and therefore remains a hypothesis which may have something in it but which cannot be tested. There have been attempts, mainly in America, to measure stress by looking at various personality types. Some may be familiar with the work done by Rosen and Freeman which divides people into Type A and Type B. Type A being the time conscious ambitious person who you might describe as being under stress and Type B being the type of person who lacks these characteristics. There is a suggestion that Type A characters have more coronary disease than Type B but it's a terribly crude approach.

There may be some very important answers but how you actually investigate these is something which still eludes us.

Q. Dr Meade said that he wouldn't really like to push men to change their lifestyles because the outcome wouldn't help many people. That is completely contrary to the Health Education Council's 'Look After Yourself!' campaign which is trying to get people to change their lifestyles even if it does only improve the outlook for a few people.

A. Dr Meade

I go along with the idea that a lot of the things which we are hearing about now may make people feel better. I think that the right weight for height is certainly something which will make a lot of people feel a good deal better than they otherwise would. What I would say is, you have to avoid giving the impression that if you do these things everything will be alright and nobody will succumb to any of these diseases prematurely. I don't think the evidence justifies such action. The evidence for example that if you lower blood cholesterol levels, by whatever means, you will prevent some cases of coronary disease which would otherwise have occurred is unsubstantiated. Some will occur in spite of that and a lot of people will do whatever it is you advise them to do when they don't actually need to. It's a question of getting the balance right between the sort of advice which we were hearing about in the campaign on the one hand but at the same time avoiding the implication that it is a panacea for all the common diseases that we are concerned with; because it's not.

COMMENT FROM MARY DISSELDUFF: DHSS

A plea for caution. I get very frightened at the thought of radical change. The British diet may not be perfect but it has supported a reasonable population for a very long time. I do not want to sound traditionalist and say no change at all, but dietary changes, either deficiencies or interactions between our food components do not manifest themselves immediately, so it's going to be the next generation before anyone sees the effects of radical change. We have enough evidence over recent years of previously unknown nutrients, Vitamin D in breast milk which was only identified as an active component within the last few years, but there is a vast area of the unknown and this worries me. I would suggest that change should be based on facts and that it should be slow not radical.